My Life at the Gym

My Life at the Gym

Feminist Perspectives on Community through the Body

Edited by
JO MALIN

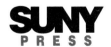

Published by State University of New York Press, Albany

For information, contact State University of New York Press, Albany, NY
www.sunypress.edu

Production by Diane Ganeles
Marketing by Michael Campochiaro

Library of Congress Cataloging-in-Publication Data

My life at the gym : feminist perspectives on community through the body / edited by Jo Malin.
    p. cm.
  Includes bibliographical references and index.
  ISBN 978-1-4384-2943-4 (hardcover : alk. paper)
  ISBN 978-1-4384-2944-1 (pbk. : alk. paper)
  1. Feminism.   2. Exercise for women—Psychological aspects.   3. Dance for women—Psychological aspects.   I. Malin, Jo, 1942–

HQ1154.M934 2010
613.71082—dc22   2009012934

10 9 8 7 6 5 4 3 2 1

Contents

List of Figures   vii

Acknowledgments   ix

Introduction   1
  Jo Malin

PART 1   THE DANCE

Chapter 1   An Elegy for Dancing   19
  Christina Pugh

Chapter 2   Kaleidoscope Dances   31
  Anne Mamary

Chapter 3   From Ballet to Boxing: The Evolution of a
Female Athlete   43
  Susan Young

Chapter 4   The Women's Dance   61
  Virginia Corrie-Cozart

PART 2   THE GYM, WEIGHT ROOM, STUDIO, AND POOL

Chapter 5   You Spin Me Right Round, Baby: Resistance,
Potential, and Feminist Pedagogy in Indoor Cycling   65
  Kristine Newhall

Chapter 6   Beyond the Lone Images of the Superhuman
Strongwoman and Well-Built Bombshell toward a
New Communal Vision of Muscular Women   79
  Jacqueline Brady

Chapter 7   Enduring Images   91
  Catherine Houser

Chapter 8   The Gymnastics Group   95
  Marcia Woodard

Chapter 9   Gym Interrupted   101
  Myrl Coulter

Chapter 10   Naked Truth   111
  Lynn Z. Bloom

Chapter 11   Women's Yoga: A Multigenre Meditation
on Language and the Body   117
  Victoria Boynton

PART 3   ON THE ROAD, THE SLOPES, AND THE LAKE

Chapter 12   "Messing about in Boats": Rowing as
l'Écriture Féminine   125
  Shannon Smith

Chapter 13   Women Who Ski with Dogs   135
  Grace D'Alo

Chapter 14   If These Roads Could Talk: Life as a
Woman on the Run   145
  Wendy Walter-Bailey

Chapter 15   Walking Is an Exercise in Friendship   151
  Marlene Jensen

Chapter 16   Marathon   155
  Beth Widmaier Capo

List of Contributors   157

Index   161

Figures

2.1   Amy Wieber. *B. F. Harridans, Cooperstown, 2004*   32

2.2   Amy Wieber. *B. F. Harridans, Cooperstown, 2004*   33

2.3   Amy Wieber. *B. F. Harridans, Cooperstown, 2004*   36

2.4   Amy Wieber. *B. F. Harridans, Cooperstown, 2004*   38

2.5   Amy Wieber. *B. F. Harridans, Cooperstown, 2004*   41

13.1 Patricia Wallach Keough. *Women Who Ski with Dogs*   142

Acknowledgments

I want first to thank all of my family members and friends who continue to believe in me as a writer and scholar. In particular Victoria Boynton is an invaluable personal and professional friend who keeps me on the writing path. I am indebted to the faculty and staff, especially Interim Dean Susan Strehle, of the School of Education of the State University of New York at Binghamton for sustained support of this project. I am especially grateful to the contributors to this volume, who share my commitment to telling the stories of "women at the gym." However, the idea for and the work of this book is most dependent on my bonds with the women I "work out" with at Shamrock Athletic Center and the inspiration I derive from the classes taught by my favorite instructors: Christine, Karen, Marcia, and Rose.

Anne Mamary's "Kaleidoscope Dances," along with photographs by Amy Wieber, was originally published in *International Studies in Philosophy* 37:1 (2005). "The Women's Dance," a poem by Virginia Corrie-Cozart, first appeared in 1991 in *Calayx, A Journal of Art and Literature by Women*.

Introduction

Jo Malin

I've lived for a long time with one kind of strength. Now I've developed a taste for another, for power and for perspiration. And I am not alone.

—Anna Quindlen, "The Irony of Iron"

As I was completing my work on the *Encyclopedia of Women's Auto-biography* with my co-editor and dear friend Victoria Boynton, I began thinking about this collection of women's life narratives that would describe and reveal the writers' participation in feminist-influenced communities that are grounded in bodywork and quietly exist at local gyms, fitness centers, and community pools; in dance or yoga studios and at skating rinks; and on neighborhood streets and mountainous hiking trails. At the end of each of those hectic days, as I do on most workdays, I would eagerly look forward to lifting weights or doing aerobics with my women friends at the gym, women who form a warm and sweaty community. However, at no time did I bring these two experiences together, that is, consider adding a topic entry or entries to the encyclopedia that would honor or privilege this equally important part of my life. Why didn't we have entries such as women's sports narratives, exercise diaries and journals, or memoirs of the gym? Why did we, as editors and also subjects of our own personal narratives and poetry, not see these particular types of stories of the body as important parts of women's life narratives and their autobiographical subjectivity? The life-writing texts by women that do exist mostly describe the lives of near-professional athletes, dancers, or competitors on collegiate athletic teams, written since the passage of Title IX of the Education Amendments of 1972 drastically changed sports for young women by focusing attention and funding on their pursuits in sports.[1]

Very often, my own workouts are the best part of my day. As soon as I sit down at my desk in the morning, my muscles are poised for my class at the end of the day. By mid-afternoon, I can't wait to get there; my body craves the exercise. And, finally, at the end of the workday when I leave my office, I'm humming some of the tunes my favorite class instructors play. The moment I enter the gym, I breathe differently, wear a different expression on my face that matches my comfortable gym shorts, T-shirt, and sneakers. I eagerly anticipate the movement, the burn, the "play" of it. I also look forward to the feeling of shared enjoyment among the women I work out with and the teachers who have become models and mentors for me and my bodywork.

Somewhere along the line of my nonlinear career and "life," my work as a writer and an editor became the close companion to *my life at the gym.* As I sit at my keyboard and do my most abstract thinking, my body provides a simple, undeniable foundation for the work. If I ignore its muscles and bones for too long, I start to feel stiff and sore as well as isolated with my thoughts. I miss the muscle sensations, the body *work* but also my companions in *my life at the gym.* We are there to *work out* and to feel the results of the workout in the following days. Yet amid this physical working is a pure sense of play, the fun of throwing off professional identity for that short time with the women who move in and out of the communal space at my gym.

Susan Bordo published in 1993 *Unbearable Weight: Feminism, Western Culture, and the Body.* Following more than a decade after Kim Chernin's *The Obsession: Reflections on the Tyranny of Slenderness,* Bordo focused the attention of feminist theory and criticism on a deep cultural fear of women's power in Western society and the growing evidence of eating disorders associated with an ever-shrinking ideal of female beauty. Bordo's study drew irrefutable parallels between these two forces: as women gain power, expectations for feminine beauty and the pressures for women to be ever thinner increase. Today, however, women are actually growing larger, and "starving to be thin" eating disorders affect a very small minority of women in developed nations. Most current studies show that the occurrence of anorexia in adolescents is only 1 percent and that bulimia, although more secret, can be estimated at 4 percent. Despite Bordo's brilliant work and her predictions, women are not getting smaller. We have in fact grown ever larger since 1993.

The problem of obesity is at crisis levels in the West and spreading to the less developed nations of the world. Women today face a shocking future in which our daughters may not live even as long as we do. Yet recognizing this crisis, along with an acute awareness, as feminists, of the cultural messages women are bombarded with that narrowly define acceptable feminine body image and that may govern our attempts at body "work," many women are finding comfortable and healthful spaces that allow them to take care of the physical needs of their bodies for some form of exercise. Throughout our lives and especially as we age, physical exercise is essential for our hearts, bones, muscles, and mental health. This book focuses on the found spaces for this activity as places of community with other women. Though very diverse, the essays, personal narratives, and poems all portray everyday lives in which women have found ways to move their bodies and to gain meaning from the sites of this movement and the companions with whom they move. Many of the selections contain emerging voices revealing thoughts that may not always find their way into scholarship.

The feminist acceptance of wisdom in *The Tyranny of Slenderness* and *Unbearable Weight* and the acute consciousness of why we as women seek to be small and slender may have also ushered in the sometimes dangerous illusion that healthful exercise is unfeminist and may, even today, cause some feminists to hide their regular "gym" attendance or, at a minimum, segregate it from their activism and scholarship. The worlds of their regular exercise and their feminist theoretical writing have not overlapped unless they are sport or dance theorists. Despite this segregation of experience, there is a quiet and underground movement of women who have made the healthful routine of exercise a very important part of their lives. Many of us are participants in a steady, even daily, routine that includes membership in a "gym" culture, often shared with a community of women that can be found in multiple sites: dance studios, weight rooms, swimming pools, ski slopes, lakes, and even streets and sidewalks.

What makes this trend and the narratives of it so important is that today, at the start of the twenty-first century, women can no longer ignore the effects of an inactive lifestyle. A modern life that does not include regular exercise predisposes one to cancer, heart disease, high blood pressure, diabetes, stroke, and even depression.

Science has shown that the brain as well as the body is influenced by increasing the heart rate in aerobic activity. In her article "Fitness Is a Feminist Issue," Tara Brabason sees "fitness-based communities of women as a positive force" and draws particular attention to the benefits of exercise to the strength of women's bones:

> The health situation has grown so problematic that any movement should be rewarded and encouraged. . . . For women, this movement is particularly important. It has been shown in a study of 10,000 that active women were 36 per cent [sic] less likely to break a hip in later years than the inactive. (Brabason 2006, 68, 72)

Writing for the Associated Press on February 20, 2008, Marilynn Marchione described a study of strokes among middle-age women in the United States. She concludes: "Women's waistlines are nearly two inches bigger than they were a decade earlier, and that bulge corresponds with an increase in strokes" (1).[2]

The contributors to this collection, many of whom are academics and writers, describe ways in which inclusion of regular physical exercise in their otherwise cerebral lives is enriching and very basic to their heath and their identities as aware feminists. They have also found a sense of community with those with whom they exercise, change in locker rooms, and nurse sore muscles throughout their life spans. Their ages range from twenty-nine through seventy-five, and the volume thus speaks to the possibilities of fitness and exercise throughout the aging process.

The voices in this book may appear tentative to some and perhaps they are. Is this because our culture trivializes women's physical activity as leisure, while men who "work out" are participating in sport? Or because our culture also trivializes women's physical activity as only associated with diet/weight loss and appearance? The writers here are moving for the sake of their health and longevity but also for the joy and pleasure of kinetic engagement and the enjoyment of feeling their bodies grow stronger, bigger, and more muscular.

Also, many are voices of women over forty for whom life before Title IX included elementary and secondary schools with meager and poorly funded opportunities to participate in physical activity. This history of prejudice is also reflected in the fact that many write about and have participated only in dance, running, or swimming, all activities that require less funding than football, for example.

Feminist consciousness of the body is not what it was in 1993 when Bordo's important book was published. Despite more than a decade of our awareness of the constricting of the female body to a young and slender anorexic ideal, those of us who write of women and women's lives have mediated these limited cultural norms with the realities of our own need for physical activity and our enjoyment of it. Even Bordo told her reader that through a national weight loss program she had achieved a major weight loss. She defends this loss as perhaps hypocritical, given her scholarship:

> In 1990, I lost twenty-five pounds through a national weight-loss program, a choice that some of my colleagues viewed as inconsistent and even hypocritical, given my work. But in my view, feminist cultural criticism is not a blueprint for the conduct of personal life. . . . Its goal is edification and understanding, enhanced *consciousness* of the power, complexity, and *systemic* nature of culture; . . . simply becoming *more conscious* is a tremendous achievement. (Bordo 1993, 30, emphases in original)

As feminist scholars mostly in the fields of literature and women's studies, we all are women with bodies that need the exercise that will help us thrive and even live longer. In addition, those who ignore exercise not only lose an avenue to improving or sustaining health but also one for enjoyment and community.

I came to this community at my gym late in life. As part of my evolution as a feminist, I started to explore this traditional masculine space as a middle-age woman. I didn't move into it directly, through sports or through youthful recreational pursuits. I entered, rather, through the dance studio. When I was five years old, my mother took me to my first dance lesson. The class included tap and ballet lessons and was made up entirely of little girls dressed in black leotards, transported there by our mothers. I don't remember the day of the first class or how I felt. I do know, today, that it was the beginning of my lifelong identity as a dancer. This first dance experience was also my first membership in a community of women and girls, but I was far too young to understand the uniqueness and value of its female-centered character, as well as the fact that it was an expected space for many young girls. In retrospect, I can see a lot about both the wonders of a female-centered community and the downside—the "charm and grace" that dance purports to teach girls, the constructed nature of the feminine in dance, and the emphasis on the body as object, in this experience.

By age twelve, I came to the painful conclusion that I did not have the talent to be a professional ballerina, though I knew I was a dancer. I enrolled in a ballroom dance class at my school. It was for both boys and girls and met on Saturday nights and fulfilled my pre-adolescent need for more heterosexually-based dance. I also started going to school dances. In high school, I continued "social dancing" and added modern dance to my life. I was so accustomed to the structure and choreography of tap and ballet that I found it challenging to step outside the moves I knew and begin creating with any freshness in modern dance. But I was a dancer and loved this *women's* community of dance class as I did as a younger girl. In college I continued with this form of movement and added synchronized swimming, which felt a lot like dancing. These were also classes that attracted only women. After college, as a young wife and mother, international folk dancing absorbed some of my attention, and eventually English and American country dancing became my favorites. Since that time, I've added Cotswold Morris dancing and step aerobics to my repertoire.

For sixteen years, I have been a member of a women's Morris team. Morris dancing is a very old English traditional dance related to fertility and good fortune. Membership on my team, the B. F. Harridans, means weekly practices, which are demanding and strenuous, and performances at public festivals and local events in the spring and summer. This dancing on the team also provides an identity that coalesces around physical activity and women's community. All of these years of varied dancing have been central to my identity as a woman, among other like-minded women, devoted to female physicality.

My first experience at an actual gym or "fitness club" began about eighteen years ago. I started with classes in basic and then "step" aerobics. Brief sessions of lifting free weights also were part of these classes. I now go to my gym five or six days a week, depending on my Morris practice schedule. I attend classes rather than use the treadmills or other equipment. Sometimes I attend step aerobics classes, but more and more I choose "PowerFit," which is a group weight-lifting session using barbells and dumbbells. I am finding it extremely satisfying to be able to lift heavier and heavier weights and to watch and feel my muscles growing. The instructors obviously work very hard at creating a supportive environment, and the other students are almost always women. These classes provide a model of a feminist community based on physical exercise, as does my Morris dancing.

I have written articles and books as a feminist literary scholar, especially in the area of women's autobiography. I also write grant proposals and work in a grant-supported university position. The subject of my writing has never been about my gym and my fitness and this community of women with whom I move. Up until now, the gym simply has been where I go at the end of my work and writing days and also during my weekends. As I turn my attention to theorizing this experience, the muscle work and the community, I've entered a body of feminist critique that addresses women and sport, women and fitness, and women and recreation. The essays and poems brought together in this book begin to describe an experience of community and connection that women build and have built through their bodies and the often happy work of keeping them in motion.

Lynda Johnston wrote in 1998, "Historically, entry by women into gyms—an exclusively male environment—was not easily achieved" (250). The high school experience I had with "physical education" did little to make me feel welcome in the world of the gym and the world of women's sports. I always felt uneasy and inadequate on the court or in the field and with a ball in my hands. The pool was a welcome milieu, but even there I moved away from team competition and toward water safety classes and synchronized swimming rather than competition. I'm sure that larger cultural forces in the pre-Title IX world I grew up in prevented me from even dreaming about athletics as a path. In fact, I didn't hold a dumbbell or a barbell in my hands until ten years ago. My preference for the more "feminine" movement of dance was reinforced at every turn.

Now that I am in the gym, though interestingly I still choose the group exercise studio within the gym, I am there so frequently that it has become almost a second home to me. Shari Dworkin calls it her second home in her article "A Woman's Place is in the . . . Cardiovascular Room?? Gender Relations, the Body, and the Gym" (2003, 135). It can also be described as a "third place," neither home nor work, a community space that mediates the gap between the two (Trebay 2006, 1). In *The Great Good Place*, Ray Oldenburg bemoans the loss of neighborhood diners or general stores where one is known and welcomed among old friends in an easy, ongoing community. I share my third place mostly with women. This gym space has the intimate feeling associated with sharing the body and its many "stories"—tales of injury, illness, food, and the changes of age. The space is still a fragile, new space of feminist support for me and for many of the women who exercise there and share the connection of moving together.

This book focuses on some of the spaces feminists have found for exercise, as places of community with other women. Though very diverse, the essays, personal narratives, and poems all portray everyday lives in which women have found ways to move their bodies and to gain meaning from the sites of this movement and the companions with whom they move. The dialogue they engage in with other women through their bodies is clearly very meaningful. The contributors' feminist, and mostly scholarly, prisms inform their gym and studio experiences. "The gym" is representative not only of the dance studio but of the pool, the weight room, and the skating rink. Women also take their gym experiences outside and on the road, the lake, and the slopes.

Part 1 of *My Life at the Gym* is called "The Dance," and thus this collection begins where I began my life at the gym—in the dance studio. My own participation in dance, from ballet to ballroom to Morris, has always crossed the line between art and athletics. The contributors in this section dance on that line and around it in a complicated verbal narrative that is quite similar to choreography. The complicated issue of body size and shape in dance has been treated in feminist criticism very thoroughly and is not overlooked in this section. Young girls (and boys), particularly those who study ballet and gymnastics, are subjected to pressures that may lead to eating disorders.

In chapter 1, "An Elegy for Dancing," Christina Pugh describes the contrast between the kind of thinking she does while dancing and the thinking she does when she swims laps or plods ahead on a treadmill. Her essay is also an elegy for that part of her life lived as a dancer and her loss of that identity and community because of a painful back condition. She describes the studio in physical, evocative language. In her words, "I had dancing in the blood." Yet she goes past the physical to write of what she misses most, which is the experience of movement along with using that part of her brain that used to "light up" with complete Heideggerean presence. She writes that when she swims laps she cannot escape from her "self," the self that is identified with her work: "As I swim laps, I am certainly 'working out,' in the common parlance; but I am working out my schedule, my responsibilities, my preoccupations." In the dance studio she was able to escape from this self because complete kinesthetic engagement was required. Also, her description of the feeling that some dancers have—"if we simply keep up the practice, we can do it all our lives"—will seem quite accurate in its simplistic yet clearly flawed logic to anyone who loves to dance. Pugh concludes with a conversation at an artist's colony with an athlete who has similar chronic pain problems. This talk and the very act of writing her elegy bring her some perspective and self-consolation.

In chapter 2, "Kaleidoscope Dances," Anne Mamary describes these as a "set" of several short dances of different tempi, timbres, rhythms, textures, and feels. It grows out of her experience as a member of a women's Morris dance team and is structured around lyrics of traditional English folk tunes. Her contribution, she writes, "dances into being bodies kinetic, audacious, and libidinous; it sets in motion a poetic vision, one that takes space yet makes freedom." Her "set" of dances is accompanied by photographs of the B. F. Harridans Morris team.

Susan Young, in chapter 3, "From Ballet to Boxing: The Evolution of a Female Athlete," examines her journey from professional ballet dancer to professional figure skater to novice boxer. The three identities coincide with three decades of her adult life and, as such, they represent distinct phases in her eventual rejection of traditional and current ideologies defining female physicality. She also describes her gradual understanding that escaping body-image tyranny is not a matter of revelation but evolution. For her, a crucial factor in this evolutionary process was the presence and encouragement of other women—from ice-dancing coaches to personal trainers—who presented her with "dazzling, powerful models of female athleticism and physical strength."

Young also reflects on the profound ways in which her evolution as a woman athlete has strengthened her connection to other women outside of the studio, rink, and gym. She then addresses the more general issue of athletic empowerment for women, from both personal experiential and broader sociological perspectives.

Part 1 concludes with Virginia Corrie-Cozart's poem in chapter 4, "The Women's Dance." The poem grew out of the experience of attending her stepson's wedding and remembering or conjuring up all the myths and images of women that have evolved for such events. Women's historical community, movement, and physicality are celebrated during the brief time of the "ladies dance" that sets the bride and the women at the wedding apart from the groom and the male guests.

In part 2, "The Gym, Weight Room, Studio, and Pool," six essays plus a prose and poetic "piece" explore and theorize within these varied interior spaces where women exercise their bodies and find community. In chapter 5, "You Spin Me Right Round, Baby: Resistance, Potential, and Feminist Pedagogy in Indoor Cycling," Kristine Newhall writes that she became an avid indoor cyclist or "spinner" because she likes many aspects of the workout. However, when she first started, she often found the instructor's comments or the lyrics of the music sexist and degrading. Her eventual defense was to become an instructor herself instead of continuing to work out while attempting to ignore the musical and vocal messages about how she should eat, exercise, and just *be* a woman. During her first year as a spinning instructor, she was also engaged in research on feminist pedagogy and sports studies. She became acutely aware of alternate methods to encourage her students: emphasizing the individual challenge over any aesthetic result and carefully choosing her playlist to avoid songs that reference the idealized female body of mass media.

Newhall's essay makes use of feminist pedagogy, sports scholarship on group exercise and empowerment, cultural theory on gender and space, and personal narrative to explore how group exercise instructors can begin to dismantle gender norms of health and fitness. Newhall concludes that instructors have the potential for disruption when they create an environment and a workout that attempt to counter the newly hegemonic ideal of the toned, but not bulky, female musculature.

In chapter 6, "Beyond the Lone Images of the Superhuman Strongwoman and the Well-Built Bombshell toward a New Communal Vision of Muscular Women," a sociohistorical analysis of the development of women's bodybuilding in America, Jacqueline Brady looks skeptically at the current celebration of the muscular female. She argues that in elevating these strong women to the status of rugged individuals and feminist icons, our culture has created representations that erase the sometimes unhealthy work that goes into the making of such bodies. But even more unfortunately, these celebrations of individuated muscular bodies remove the female bodybuilder from her community of other women bodybuilders. In so doing, they take her out of the communal space of the gym where she actually operates most of the time and where she engages in a process of female community formation that can lead to real social change.

Brady writes that women's bodybuilding actually brings together a variety of women in small groups for an activity based on changing the body and, more generally, on changing cultural styles of self-representation—changing the ways women see themselves and the ways the general culture sees women. She feels that it is this communal aspect of physical and psychological transformation that holds out the hope of creating new meanings. As an example she sees some of the more promising results of female strength not in the depictions of lone women flexing their muscles but in the vigorous collective efforts of women using sport as a context for social change in efforts such as a walk to raise funds for breast cancer research.

Catherine Houser, in chapter 7, "Enduring Images," writes of the older women she looks to at her gym as models for aging instead of unrealistic media images but also because she lost her "lifelong model for perseverance and endurance" when her mother died shortly after Houser turned forty. In her personal narrative here she describes the loosely knit community of women at her gym who come together in the early morning hours. Many are in their seventies and eighties and of the age her mother would have been today. She writes that as an academic she is surrounded by examples of how to go through her fifties and sixties professionally but, as Houser says, "in the physical world those powerful, positive images have been more difficult to come by—until I began noticing those women at my gym." She narrates an experience of easy community where she is constantly learning how to age from the women she works out with.

Marcia Woodard's humorous personal essay "The Gymnastics Group," chapter 8, begins with her elementary school experience of "failing" at tumbling. She draws in the reader with her vivid descriptions of childhood physical education classes that are funny and very accurate for many women. She writes of finally finding a measure of athletic success in high school on the cross-country team, where her ability to run "slow and steady" put her at an advantage.

Woodard's contribution ends with her current, fifty-year-old athletic pursuit of leisurely walking around Greenlake in Seattle, where she feels comfortable and at home. She meets her friends there, and the focus is "more social than sweat." They walk and talk, and she participates in a supportive women's community based on physical exercise. What she finds in this community is central to the theme of the entire collection and echoes all of the other voices, as they circle around issues of women's health and the escape from the centuries-old constraints of daintiness, with the help of like-minded others.

In chapter 9, "Gym Interrupted," Myrl Coulter describes herself as a veteran of hundreds of workout classes who possesses a strange assortment of exercise clothing that mostly lies hidden in the dark recesses of her closet. Her humorous essay tells the tale of twenty-five years of experience at various gyms and fitness centers with short bursts of energetic participation and long interruptions. Motivation is her constant challenge, and she writes of a struggle to stay engaged. Finally, though, the "gym women" always draw her back, and at the end of the essay she is comfortable with her trips to the gym to walk on the treadmill.

Lynn Z. Bloom's "Naked Truth," chapter 10, describes her own exercise experience, which is without the interruptions that Coulter struggles with. It is a series of short vignettes connected by the daily rhythms of her lap swimming and the conversations that literally come to the surface and continue in the locker room. This watery ritual has come to be one of the most important and unchanging elements of Bloom's life. She writes of the use of the simple query "How are you?" and the attendant responses, in this space, which often reveal feelings of nakedness not experienced in the other spaces of daily life. She calls her friends from the pool "veterans of the deep."

Part 2 concludes with Victoria Boynton's "Women's Yoga: A Multigenre Meditation on Language and the Body," chapter 11. In her piece, she uses meditative prose, academic reflection, and poetry to discuss how the physical exercises of yoga change the relation of the mind and body. Boynton asserts that these ancient yoga practices can alleviate the contemporary focus on "mentality" and the resulting stress in women's lives. She argues that in this physical practice, thought takes on a different character, relieving the taxed mind of its usual overactivity. The yoga studio space in which hyperthought falls away through exercise serves as both a material locale and a metaphor of containment and protection for "losing one's mind," so to speak. Boynton's weaving of genre parallels the way the mind shifts gears as the body comes into focus through yoga practice in a safe studio space.

Part 3, "On the Road, the Slopes, and the Lake," begins with Shannon Smith's " 'Messing about in Boats': Rowing as *l'Écriture Féminine*," chapter 12. She takes part of her title from Kenneth Grahame's Edwardian children's novel *The Wind in the Willows* (1933 [1908]). In it, the self-assured character Rat sings the praises of sculling to his riverbank friend, Mole: "Believe me, my young friend, there is *nothing*—absolutely nothing—half so much worth doing as simply messing about in boats" (8, emphasis in original). She compares this description of a feeling of movement free from the linear constraints of an origin and a destination to Hélène Cixous's description of *l'écriture féminine*, a mode of creative expression that contrasts with the standard model of "male writing."

Smith's essay originates in her experience of a conscious adoption of this model by her women's crew team composed of faculty and graduate students from the Department of English at Queen's University who also engage in collaborative writing. She explores the ways in which these models challenge both the Romantic ideal of the individual author and the archetype of the male athlete.

Chapter 13, "Women Who Ski with Dogs," by Grace D'Alo, chronicles an annual trip over the President's Day holiday weekend in February by eight to twelve female friends, between fifty and sixty years old. As they have for twelve years, the women leave their homes and jobs in Carlisle, Pennsylvania, and drive to a cabin in Ontario, where they relish the opportunities inherent in a frozen environment. They ski, often with their dogs, skate, build fires, cook, and talk for four days. D'Alo writes: "Despite ankle reconstructions, knee replacements, and frozen shoulders we have nurtured our physical selves without competitiveness or pressure." Her personal narrative, accompanied by a copy of a painting of the same name, by Patricia Walach Keough, details this unusual annual trip that binds these women together.

Wendy Walter-Bailey, in chapter 14, "If These Roads Could Talk: Life as a Woman on the Run," describes herself as a lifelong athlete who began running competitively in sixth grade. But here she writes about the change in this life-of-running when she decided to join a women's running group to train for a half marathon. She says, "My life changed when I started running with women." She describes a feminist fitness community that she has found to be even more powerful than the feminist scholarly community she discovered earlier as an academic. Her narrative echoes some of the previous tellings in this collection in that it extols the experience of finding a women's community through an exercise choice. She writes, "Running is not a glamorous sport, and the hours on the road often elicit the deepest secrets."

Marlene Jensen is a newspaper columnist and her contribution, chapter 15, "Walking Is an Exercise in Friendship," began as a column about her walking group, the Holly Hill Hiking Group. Here she chronicles her walking experience with women in her suburban Upstate New York neighborhood. For them, walking is "the basis, backdrop, and cement of their friendship." When I contacted her about including her column, she told me then that she was leaving my area and that saying good-bye to the women she walks with was proving to be very difficult. I asked her to extend the column and bring it up to date after she moved. Her subsequent essay tells the story of that move and her relationship to the women in her old and new walking groups. She writes, "Walking alone is exercise. Walking with friends, especially women friends, can be an enriching and transforming experience."

The final contribution in part 3 is the poem "Marathon," chapter 16, by Beth Widmaier Capo. It describes the process of training for and running a marathon with a friend. Capo's poem reaches toward the personal experience of sharing a physical and an emotional connection with another woman through an athletic act. She writes, "Should we look at this distance, this race run, as summarizing our lives?" and in this line, perhaps, gestures toward the meaning of the sharing of physical exercise among women in all of the essays and poems in this volume.

My Life at the Gym brings together women's narratives, meaningful life narratives that need to be heard as part of a feminist project to describe and deconstruct the lives of women today. Scholars from the humanities, education, law, and women's and literary theory, as well as poets, writers, and visual artists, have sought and are finding meaning and community in diverse sites of physical movement and fitness: gyms, dance studios, skating rinks, boxing rings, and more. Their contributions are multidimensional and diverse and can speak to many other women who seek health and long life in the twenty-first century.

Notes

1. An excellent example of a competitive female athlete's autobiographical text is Leslie Heywood's *Pretty Good for a Girl: An Athlete's Story* (Minneapolis: University of Minnesota Press, 2000).

2. Led by Amytis Towfighi, M.D., at the University of Southern California at Los Angeles, the study used the National Health and Nutrition Surveys for the period 1999–2004 and compared the data to the previous survey from the period 1988–1994.

Works Cited

Brabason, Tara. 2006. "Fitness Is a Feminist Issue." *Australian Feminist Studies* 21:49 (March): 65–83.

Bordo, Susan. 1993. *Unbearable Weight: Feminism, Western Culture, and the Body.* Berkeley: University of California Press.

Chernin, Kim. 1981. *The Obsession: Reflections on the Tyranny of Slenderness.* New York: Harper & Row.

Dworkin, Shari L. 2003. "A Woman's Place is in the . . . Cardiovascular Room?? Gender Relations, the Body, and the Gym." In *Athletic Intruders: Ethnographic Research on Women, Culture, and Exercise*, ed. Anne Bolin and Jane Granskog, 131–58. Albany: State University of New York Press.

Grahame, Kenneth. 1933 [1908]. *The Wind in the Willows.* New York: Charles Scribner's Sons.

Johnston, Lynda. 1998. "Reading the Sexed Bodies and Spaces of Gyms." In *Places through the Body*, ed. Heidi J. Nast and Steve Pile, 244–62. London: Routledge.

Marchione, Marilynn. 2008. "Strokes among Middle-Aged Women Triple" (February 20). http://www.nytimes.com/aponline/us/AP-Obesity-Strokes.html, accessed February 21, 2008.

Oldenburg, Ray. 1999. *The Great Good Place: Cafés, Coffee Shops, Bookstores, Bars, Hair Salons, and Other Hangouts at the Heart of a Community*. New York: Marlowe & Co.

Quindlen, Anna. 1997. "The Irony of Iron." http://www.sportsillustrated. cnn.com/features/1997/womenmag/essay.html, accessed February 24, 2006.

Trebay, Guy. 2006. "24-Hour Sweaty People." *New York Times*, May 21, final ed., sec. 9, p. 1.

Part 1

■

The Dance

1

An Elegy for Dancing

Christina Pugh

> In the modern sense of the term, the elegy is a short poem, usually formal or ceremonious in tone and diction, occasioned by the death of a person. Unlike the dirge, threnody, obsequy, and other forms of pure lament or memorial, however, and more expansive than the epitaph, the elegy frequently includes a movement from expressed sorrow toward consolation.
>
> —*New Princeton Encyclopedia of Poetry and Poetics*

Is it possible to write an elegy in prose? What about an allegorical elegy—an elegy for an aspect of the self that has been lost, or that remains in regression or remission? This essay—this *attempt*, to paraphrase the French verb *essayer*—will try to do both of those things: to enact a prose elegy for a dancing self, replete with some small measure of sorrow and a gesture toward self-consolation, as suggested in my epigraph's definition. For I no longer dance, due to the limitations of injury and chronic pain.

Up until now, it has only been in poems that I have tried to describe the kinesthetic sense of dancing (though more often than not, the poems have made use of the very specialized vocabulary of dance rather than the so-called "experience" of it). And by virtue of its very genre, a poem may have what Lucie Brock-Broido has called an autistic quality: "I think of poems as autistic, in the sense that they're trapped in extremity's small room—they're large thoughts that don't get to speak in prose" (1998, 146). Though we might question or quarrel with Brock-Broido's definition of *autistic*, it's clear to me that she is obliquely referring to the preverbal synergies that animate the best poems: what Kristeva discussed as the *chora*. Such energy also makes for some salutary blindness, a blindness not completely unlike that which fascinated Paul de Man. But even when I write in prose about my experience, I am likely never to see clearly when it comes to my own narrative or narratives—particularly when they concern something as quicksilver in constitution, as ephemeral in time and space as the act of dancing.

I remember the beauty of the open studio, its floor covered in a smooth black tarp called Marley. Doubled by the mirrors, it became a broad and virtual terrain—sprung so that dancers' feet were torque, traction, instrument. The quality of the floor is paramount to the dancer: too hard, and jumps become belly flops. And the risk of injury is that much greater.

When I see the empty studio in my mind's eye, I also see the margins of my modern dance classes—the moments before class began and after it ended. There was the ritual of warming up (and down): stretching knees, calves, ankles, shoulders, feet, spine. I was very flexible, as I am today; a doctor recently called it *hypermobility*. But despite my flexibility and high extensions of the leg, despite my training and devotion to class week after week, I was not a good dancer and never would be. I could not learn combinations—the stitching together of steps in muscle memory—and this failure was never reversed, even by years of study. "Either you have it or you don't," a teacher once commented on the subject; for the first time, I wondered whether there might be something constitutional or synaptic that was getting in the way of such learning, something quite different from but analogous to dyslexia, for example. (One of my best friends from college has had no sense of smell from birth. Even at the age of twenty-one, he tried to keep it a secret. He was ashamed: he thought he'd failed to learn something essential as a child.)

But I had dancing in the blood, and so I chose to struggle—or, more aptly, to remain—in a chronic state of nonmastery. My favorite teacher was fond of sinuous and very complicated combinations; according to her biographical profile, she was interested in "dynamic physicality with lyrical phrasing, and the dancer's relationship to space." I had never encountered someone so exacting and yet with so much public equanimity. She could sense the precise lay of vertebrae through a sweatshirt. She grabbed my hips and manhandled me across the Marley. She adjusted my head one inch to the left. I never spoke to her in the personal way, as Louise Glück puts it in "Birches," but her smile, in its authentic *im*personality, really could carry a whole room of bodies. I came to see the way her muscles moved, the delicate weight of the head on those shoulders, and I stored that persona somewhere for future reference.

As for myself, I talked very little before or after class. I had the requisite sharp ribs and hip bones but none of the physical or social ease of the other dancers: that garrulous love of surfaces that characterizes so many who live the life of theater and performance. One famous choreographer claimed that dancers are stupid—and, indeed, from the vantage point of choreography as a discipline, they can be as pawns on a board. In *Stupidity,* Avital Ronell calls the *dummkopf* "a creature of mimesis" and goes on to say that "the only thing that the stupid have over the smart is mechanical memory" (2003, 16–17). Movement memory, unthinking mimesis: perhaps it wasn't stupidity as such, but successful dancers really did seem to have something. I might now call it a sustained capacity for self-relinquishment: some talent for *askesis* or self-emptying, in the Christian and Bloomian sense, which allowed them to move as complexly disciplined, regulated bodies unfolding and changing in space.

Conversely, I could only see my own movement as a static sequence of flat poses: there was a vaguely Cubist quality to it all. I had the vocabulary, but I couldn't get the syntax. I was stupid, but in a different way. In Roman Jakobson's structuralist terms, I was an aphasic dancer: I had contiguity disorder, or "impairment of the ability to propositionize, or, generally speaking, to combine simpler linguistic entities into more complex units" (1971, 85). And my teacher kept adjusting the back of my neck, the spot at which the head connects to the neck: the *trapezius,* I think. *Trapeze,* then: a trapeze of consciousness unmoored from flesh. Evidently I was trying to be two places at once and not succeeding. As Peggy Phelan states so succinctly, "The body does not experience the world in the way that consciousness does" (1997, 52). The struggle to learn kinesthetically, so natural for some, was for me a continually and somatically articulated version of stage fright, since there's no faking what your feet won't do.

As graduate students, we learn how to parry, how to inhabit the position of mastery until it feels natural. When I attended talks, I heard nonanswers to questions that would continue for minutes upon eloquent minutes. That mantle of mastery was something I was learning to put on during the day; but at night it was all drum, all piano—and the hope that formulation, some sense, could come of these muscles. As in the academy, the demand was always changing:

I could practice at home, but that would never really prepare me for the new movement phrases I would have to learn the next week.

Once I heard my teacher speaking before class started. "Why is it that no matter how long I've done this, I always feel like I'm starting all over again?" she said with a small, rueful laugh. It sounded like me—or, more accurately, it sounded like what I would have said if I could. At that time, I was always looking for people who appeared to have access to what I now recognize as universal secrets, so the question stayed with me. I know this now, too, as the terribly mundane task of recreating the self every day, as we make beds: taking ourselves in hand over the blank page, for example; prodding what wants to rest on the side of the road. Of course, such work is intimately related to a writing discipline. As Ronell says, "To write is to take a retest every day" (2003, 26).

What we need in order to do this successfully, or at least consistently, is precisely the opposite of multitasking. Dance class with Sharon required nothing less than my every stray cognitive faculty—a concentration that left no room for any unengaged, or otherwise engaged, remainders of consciousness. This was fight-or-flight, a certain tincture of everyday panic. It was indeed the opposite of what Sven Birkerts has defined as our everyday state of "distracted absorption" (1994, 206) in the face of electronic media; instead, dance absorption is commensurate with his description of the *print* reader's near-beatific and bodily focus, a state of being "bathed in the energies of the book" (84). Such untranslatable concentration is necessarily operative in the reading act, as Stevens knew in "The House Was Quiet and the World Was Still":

> The words were spoken as if there was no book
> Except that the reader leaned above the page,
> Wanted to lean, wanted much most to be
> The scholar to whom his book is true. (1982, 358)

Even in its circumscription, Stevens's poem describes a bodily lancination: that *leaning* wherein the book-as-vehicle disappears so that the world becomes the reader who has become the reading act associated with askesis and, not coincidentally, with the bluntly gestural act of leaning itself: "the reader leaning late and reading there" (1982, 359). Such is the movement learning process by which we marshal our muscles into performance. Perhaps my own version of askesis didn't result in the performance I saw in other dancers, but I too forgot myself in the very effort. All of this is also intricately related to the process by which we learn poems "by heart," or the way in which we manage to put poems—and their constitutive stress patterns—into the breath and musculature of the body.

But my own story about dancing contains more than what I have just narrated here, and more than simply the struggle with movement memory. It also includes a different, concurrent narrative strand—that of my experience with the Duncan technique. In college I had taken a workshop with a dancer who taught the work of Isadora Duncan and Mary Wigman, the German expressionist choreographer. Living in Boston a few years afterwards, I had the opportunity to see the Duncan choreography again, performed by a two-dancer company called Dances by Isadora. I was transfixed by these brief dances to Chopin and Schubert pieces, performed by two women who were exquisitely attuned to each other's every glance and arm movement: one curly-haired with a round body; one slender and dimpled, with long hair. The movements were both expressive and imitative: of spring and joy, of sleeping and waking, of mythological figures such as the muses. Though neither of these women ever became famous in the dance world, I still count their performance as one of the genuinely awe-inspiring things I have seen in my life, and I was soon fortunate enough to be able to study under both of them.

What does Duncan dance entail? At the beginning of the twentieth century, Isadora Duncan positioned her new technique in opposition to balletic virtuosity, though ballet dancers are sometimes drawn to it for reasons of aesthetic and gestural similarities between the two approaches. Nevertheless, there remains an intentional check on virtuosity in the Duncan technique: the feet are not stretched to a full arch in point, the arms are not held aloft in fixed poses, and students practice simple steps such as walking and running (among others). It wasn't virtuosity as such that moved me in the performance of Dances by Isadora but instead the nuance of each movement: the grace note, the eye contact. The miracle is in the transition, as Susan Foster describes:

> ...in her *Waltzes* (ca 1913), a series of short dances to music that Duncan described as the "many faces of love," the dancer *resembles* innocent adoration, sensuous pleasure, playful flirtation, and other aspects of love during individual phrases of the dance by moving with the sustained weight of reverence, the quick lightness of play, or the shimmering undulations of sensuality. Transitional phrases between these individual sections, however, show the dancer as a person

experiencing love in its various manifestations. During these transitions the movement flows from the center of the body out to the periphery, suggesting a progressive development from "inner" feeling to "outward" form and an organic relationship between one emotional experience and the next. (Foster 1986, 71, emphasis in original)

This ritual rediscovery and treasuring of the other, dramatized recurrently in the choreography, amounts to both a romance and an ethics. As I wrote in a poem several years later, "The slowly lowered head/means more than virtuosity."

With the movements explicitly yoked to the breath in a manner that is not typical of most modern dance classes, the Duncan technique was more like meditation than dancing, though class was often vigorous. The barre exercises were the same every week: identical music, identical movements, and a stable repertoire of dances (some of which I had seen Dances by Isadora perform). The order of the day was repetition rather than combination or innovation—a world away from Sharon's class, which I took concurrently. Due to my growing familiarity with the repertoire, the Duncan technique allowed me more serenity and contemplation than I previously had been able to know in class.

The Duncan classes were not a panacea for me, insofar as they did not afford me some magic strategy to become better at learning combinations. But they did manage, incrementally, to put a different tenor of knowledge into my muscular memory, and they enabled me to start performing. The classes were about neither newness nor one person's always-changing choreographic vision. Instead, they were preservative, conservative—in the sense that they preserved a historically circumscribed, unchanged body of work (the choreography was transmitted orally from the girls Duncan adopted and taught, and then by successive generations). I say that with a bit of hesitation, since choreography is always open to interpretation, particularly the sort that lives as something of an oral tradition. And yet it is also a known quantity, particularly when one has been dancing and performing it for a while.

I brought my shyness to those studios too, but I was also aware of my own happiness in the execution. From time to time, I was very conscious that these experiences could not last forever—that I needed to be mindful of their rarity, their enormous value. And I was, sometimes; but as is the way with any genuine practice, these repertories became a way of being in the world—on some level, they became internalized and naturalized to the point of being taken for granted. You cannot imagine yourself without them. And then it is difficult to be grateful, simply because you cannot imagine yourself alive and not dancing.

The Duncan class put no limit on emotional experience; it placed a genuinely pre-Balanchine premium on expressivity. Class opens with a plié combination that conscripts the entire body, initiating the arch of the upper back from the solar plexus, the space located between the breasts. All movement in the Duncan technique is initiated from this spot, where the heart resides. The exercise ends with a precise prescription for melting the foot—toe, metatarsal, and finally the delayed heel—into the floor. The dancer thus kneads each bone incrementally, rediscovering the nexus of the foot's intricate construction. *This is where I want to be but am not. I can express the wish, but it will remain on the page as a wish: identical to any other you can imagine.*

Those italicized lines encapsulate both the difficulty of writing about "writing process" and the likely reason that "dance writing" is almost always written from the subject position of the observer—even if that observer is also concurrently a dancer. The diary of Toni Bentley, a young corps dancer in the New York City Ballet during the eighties, becomes instructive in this capacity. Trying to describe the performance of Suzanne Farrell in Balanchine's *Diamonds,* Bentley finds herself at a loss for words, or at least at a loss for the dance vocabulary that is ordinarily at her fingertips:

> Suzanne just finished another *Diamonds,* and frankly I cannot put any words on paper to describe her magnificence, her giving. I watch her face and can only think of a love she has greater than I could ever contain. She is from God's world—a direct disciple, I think. . . . I suppose the first reaction to such a sight and emotion is to define it.
>
> Isn't that what critics do? By defining and attempting to explain her we attempt, I'm sure, to submerge and put aside the sadness that her simple self evokes. She is not to be explained—she cannot be—but it is hard to bear such a sight. Surely any of our mortal words put down to explain her or describe her are absurd. (Bentley 1982, 30–31)

Bentley's sense of the necessary incommensurability of dance and writing—exemplified in her jejune yet uncannily perceptive hero worship of Farrell's performance—is a theme that continues throughout her diary: ". . . you have to be an unhappy dancer to write at all. If I were totally at peace dancing, I would have nothing to say" (1982, 133).

Certainly it is a commonplace that the phenomenology of the dancing subject resists verbal description. But if even the observer propounds the beatitude of the nonverbal—which the Bentley passage describes better, perhaps, than most—it becomes that much more difficult to parse, and to recreate through language, exactly what is lost when these experiences are no longer in the body of the dancer.

And yet one can still begin to enumerate losses—as, for example, that swept sense of body-mind expenditure that one has after dancing, particularly after a class with someone like Sharon. My own struggle with kinesthetic learning—probably because it was, of necessity, abjectly focused—purged any other thoughts that might have been in my mind during the rest of the day. And perhaps I needed to clean my mind of thoughts: not only to dance but also to write—in order to come to new discoveries in my academic work.

Everyone has a different way of accomplishing this. I had a friend who needed to watch junk TV from eleven each night until one in the morning in order to continue his writing on Heidegger and Gibson from one until dawn. But for me, television is far from a complete emptying of self: I am still there; I am the one who is watching it. Reading, particularly novelistic reading, can accomplish that emptying, as Stevens and Birkerts variously articulated—but it's also fuel and spur for my writing, thus in some way energizing and buttressing the identity of the known self in its artistic and creative ambitions. It can become, at least in part, a means to an end. For years, I've loved Roland Barthes's articulation of the phenomenon of intellectually *productive* distraction:

> To be with the one I love and to think of something else: this is how I have my best ideas, how I best invent what is necessary to my work. Likewise for the text: it produces, in me, the best pleasure if it manages to make itself heard indirectly; if, reading it, I am led to look up often, to listen to something else. (Barthes 1975, 24)

Barthes's last sentence constitutes the dilemma and joy of the poet—to whom, as Frost said, knowledge sticks like burrs. But dancing was, in most senses, disconnected from the work that comprised "my best ideas," that forged my identity in the world.

I find now that there is little escape from that self: from the one who is identified with the work. As someone who no longer takes dance classes but who "exercises," I can easily tell you the difference. As I swim laps, I am certainly "working out," in the common parlance; but

I am working out my schedule, my responsibilities, my preoccupations. The "work" is by its nature repetitive; the body understands what to do; there is no input from the mind, so it is free to go off on its usual independent peregrinations. The body is quantifiably benefited, I suppose, but there is no respite from self. There is no opportunity to engage some part of the mind differently—to light up, as it were, a different aspect of the brain. It is all numbingly familiar. The way I manage the task of it is to try to forget that I am there doing it.

Isn't this the way with nearly all of the exercise that qualifies as such for Americans today? No wonder so few of us want to do it. The ubiquitous contraption of the treadmill is also an apt metaphor for the way in which most exercise functions for us: purposeless, dutiful "spinning of wheels," from which we'll distract ourselves by any means possible (magazines, headsets, anything to trick us into thinking we're not actually using our bodies). The state of super-alert mental receptivity required in the dance class is not necessary for the sorts of physical endeavors in which we're all told to engage—in order to live longer, feel better, be a better specimen of body. Thus the exercise that we do, if we do it at all, is emphatically *non*transformative in any kind of genuinely integrative psychosomatic manner. If I have just digressed from the elegiac narrative at hand, then perhaps I have also begun to illustrate, very imperfectly, what I loved about dancing and what I miss about it now.

These days, I think a lot about mimesis in the arts. Sometimes that is indeed the only way I can think about the ambition and practice of art and my own particular place in it: not as a mimesis of the empirical world—the popular conception of Stendhal's mirror in the street—but as a sort of inescapable intertextuality that renders all of our work conservative of a prior tradition. If my poems can preserve some aspect of Donne or Dickinson in an inchoate way, then I have done my job as a necessarily belated poet, in the historical sense. But these have been my concerns for years: my dissertation was centrally focused upon issues of mimesis in the ekphrastic lyric, and I have taught in a writing program whose pedagogical model was imitation—that is, training undergraduate students to write by teaching them to imitate major poets.

The issues in dance class were, for me, very connected to these concerns. What dancers must experience, and what I experienced for years in Sharon's class, was a necessarily imperfect mimesis: we all must fall short of our teachers' movements, of our teachers' bodies. The margin for error is redefined in a dance class, in which the question becomes that of literally doing what one sees—and realizing that one cannot seamlessly approximate it, and continuing nonetheless. Perhaps this is always the fate of the nonprofessional in any artistic medium; in fact, being an amateur in some field may well give us a different and necessary lens on the field in which we are able to excel, even if we are excelling in a comparative or relative sense.

Still, it may be too simple to contrast dancing and writing for publication (to take the obvious example). My writing is something I do by myself, with no audience. I have tried to perfect it before sending it out anywhere. Let's just say that I have had innumerable hours to rehearse: to fidget with the line break, the semicolon, the comma. To mouth again the precise way in which the stress must fall before the enjambment. But in the dance studio, it was only the crowd of dancers and the present moment: no props, no crutches, no footnotes. (When I lock my locker at the pool, I'm often startled at how free I feel without my book bags and laptop; my hands are so light that I wonder how I'll accomplish anything, so unfettered.) Do I ever feel that I hit the mark with poems? Yes, I do. If I didn't, I would never send them out for publication. It may not be anyone else's mark, but it is my own, and when I have reached that mark, I know it in my ear.

Teaching writing is different, because I will never be able to replicate that feeling for students or to create it within them. I may give them assignments with mimetic components, but I can never actually create the trajectory through which they must achieve that mimesis. I can advise, but I can't enact. Strangely enough, one of the best things I can do for them is to be a version of Sharon, with her capaciousness and equanimity and energy for the art, though my eye trains lines of poems rather than of vertebrae. Dance class, more than any class in graduate school really, taught me the *persona*—not the curriculum—I would need as a shy person who wanted to teach. I learned that energy is something one can assume and, indeed, some-thing one owes to one's students. I also learned that it feeds on itself when you are doing something you love.

Though it may sound utopian, or Puritan, I do believe that we can self-create through work. When Sharon was preparing to have major surgery, her persona was indistinguishable from what it was on a normal day. I took note of that. I learned the virtues of a public persona in part by studying my dance teachers *as* teachers—their expressions, their energies, their verbal articulations—just as I studied their movements. Surely without ever intending to, Sharon had taught me an ethics of teaching—and the ethics of teaching someone who can never, constitutionally, hit the mark of what is put in front of her.

I return to the elegiac nature of this essay. We don't really want to learn lessons from what we love doing, we only want to continue doing it; and a certain strain of modern dancer believes that if we simply keep up the practice, we can do it all our lives (like Graham, like Cunningham). During a recent stay at an artists' colony, I found myself in conversation with Emily, a photographer who asked what I had been working on that day. She was interested in the topic of this essay and shared with me her own story of being forced out of competitive martial arts practice due to chronic pain when she was in her mid-thirties—quite young, according to our contemporary manner of thinking about life span.

"But you know, that's the age when people traditionally retired from competitive practice," she said. "We think we should be able to keep doing everything and don't understand anymore that we need to do different activities at different times in our lives." Now she surfs out in Rockaway, and that has steadied her. I realized that my chiropractor had said similar things to me five or seven years ago, and I had reacted with nothing but silent outrage. I wanted to dance, no matter what. But somehow in the course of writing this essay, I was able to listen to Emily differently. Perhaps writing the essay was helping me put to rest a certain part of myself. Or perhaps I wanted once again—endlessly—to turn to someone who seemed to have more wisdom than I thought I would ever have. I don't know, but that brief conversation meant a great deal to me as I was trying to put this narrative in perspective. It is hard to give up parts of the self that we have treasured, even in their failures—but a large part of living must require us to do just that.

Still, it was in dance class that I learned most viscerally the value that was to have longevity in my career: the energy, as well as the humility, of asymptotic mimesis. I try to bring both of those qualities into the classroom with my students, as we read and write poetry. I also maintain a life of the body, through swimming and stretching, in that perennial state of *hypermobility* that I have come to see as my natural element—though admittedly with less joy than in the Duncan studios. I still want to think, so unscientifically, that regions of the mind can light up, almost like Christmas trees. If there is some measure of darkness in that forest, then there can surely also still be growth.

Works Cited

Barthes, Roland. 1975. *The Pleasure of the Text*. New York: Noonday.

Bentley, Toni. 1982. *Winter Season.* New York: Random House.

Birkerts, Sven. 1994. *The Gutenberg Elegies.* New York: Ballantine.

Brock-Broido, Lucie, and Wayne Koestenbaum. 1998. "A Conversation between Lucie Brock-Broido and Wayne Koestenbaum." *Parnassus: Poetry in Review* 23:1–2: 143–65.

Foster, Susan. 1986. *Reading Dancing.* Berkeley: University of California Press.

Jakobson, Roman. 1971. "Two Aspects of Language and Two Types of Aphasic Disturbances." In *Fundamentals of Language,* ed. Roman Jakobson and Halle Morris, 69–96. The Hague: Mouton.

Phelan, Peggy. 1997. *Mourning Sex.* New York: Routledge.

Preminger, Alex, and T. V. F. Brogan, eds. 1993. *New Princeton Encyclopedia of Poetry and Poetics.* Princeton, NJ: Princeton University Press.

Ronell, Avital. 2003. *Stupidity.* Urbana: University of Illinois Press.

Stevens, Wallace. 1982. *The Collected Poems.* New York: Vintage.

2

Kaleidoscope Dances

Anne Mamary

We live in a world of signs.
But not everybody has to trade in them.

—Zadie Smith, *Autograph Man*

I. Once to Yourself

These dances, Morris dances, are ancient and new, transplanted and just born, shoved aside, forgotten, invented, resuscitated, remembered. Six women and silence frame the dance yet to begin. A wisp of hair coils across her shoulder and hankies flutter in the breeze. Six breathing, six in that moment. At her nod, the accordion breathes its fill, and the music sings once to yourself before six dancers surge into motion.

Morris dancing, its origins unknown, an organic shoot in rural England, nearly plucked out in the industrial revolution, in modernity's move to the city, to the machine-life of production, of the planet. Morris dancing red hot in my aching knees, in the arm movements beginning in the very middle of our bellies, in muscles hard as ropes. Only these bodies and accordion breathing to shape the dance, to shape the world, invented, these bodies, in the dance, in history, in movement and loss. We dance an improvised future, letting go, being cut loose, taking liberties with what was not ours, with what is as vital as the pounding of feet on pavement or the hearts in our chests.

Time was the movements of the stars and the growing of the fields turned the dance. Time was the planet and our bodies were

31

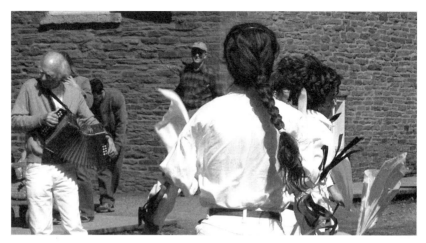

Figure 2.1. Amy Wieber. *B. F. Harridans, Cooperstown, 2004.*

dances before a cyborg future, an electric future. Not nostalgia, rather a new movement; dancing a future where our feet touch a planet not stripped of its spirit for the wealth of a few. Time will be flexible, music and dance moving together, faster now slower, pulsing to the needs of these bodies, our dances here, and those dances there, and dances I will never know there and here. Time will be.

II. "Jock O' Hazeldean"

"Jock O' Hazeldean"
Why weep ye by the tide, lady, why weep ye by the tide?
A'll wad ye tae my youngest son an ye sall be his bride
An ye sall be his bride lady sae comely tae be seen
Bit aye she lout the tears dounfaa for Jock O Hazeldean

Nou let this willfu grief be dune an dry those cheeks sae pale
Young Frank is chief of Erthington an Lord O Langleydale
His step is first in peacefu haa his sword in battle keen
Bit aye she lout the tears dounfaa for Jock O Hazeldean

A coat o gowd ye sallnae lack nor kaim tae bind your hair
Nor mettled hound nor managed hawk nor palfrey fresh an
    fair
An you, the foremaist o them aa sall ride, our forest queen
Bit aye she lout the tears dounfaa for Jock O Hazeldean

The kirk was deckt at mornintide, the tapers glimmert fair
The priest an bridegroum wait the bride an dame an knight
   were there
They searcht for her in bower an haa the lady wisnae seen
She's owre the border an awa wi Jock O Hazeldean

Six breathing. Six standing, waiting. Silence, but the dance has already begun. Buttons and reeds, accordion breathing, she gives the sign, a wave of the hand, animation. Melancholy refrain.

Six women embody one dance. In one dance, six women move, each in her own way. Tendons and muscles tight, tendons and muscles supple, tendons and muscles held girlishly, held uniquely, each a gift of nature and each unfolding a life's maps.

From the first days of our life a narrative begins whose end we already know. With our narratives we postpone the end by making some touching-up to childhood, love and nature while poetry reinvents us to the bones and star dust. Our body is a book of stories: libidinal body, body of suffering, body of tenderness, tempestuous body, lost and found again body as an origin (Brossard 1996, 6).

Six dance a woman weeping by the water, weeping at the bitterness of her body a token of exchange, her father and her bridegroom bargaining, offering her a place in exchange for her woman's body. Six dance her grief in the traditions of church and family, her grief at being bought and sold, at the body of suffering while she aches for her love, for her freedom, for tempestuous reinvention of her life's narrative.

Two sidestep, hankies an embrace across distance, and linger, linger in her grief. Two caper energetically, calf muscles and verve. Two nearly collide, pass at the last moment; two dance low to highlight

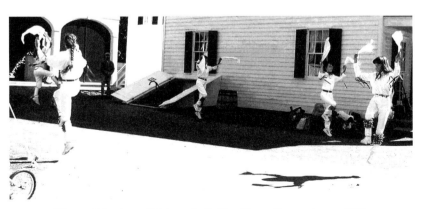

Figure 2.2. Amy Wieber. *B. F. Harridans, Cooperstown, 2004.*

one push at the start of each phrase. Two dance a smile in the air as the world vanishes but for two dancers and sustaining melody.

Six dance a full circle, six embody tenderness, embody struggle, embody poetry, six lives embodied in a kaleidoscopic dance. Six trace the patterns of centuries and there make patterns only imagined. Six dance round and round her grief over nature as an excuse for bondage. Six dance.

Six dance her freedom to an old tune, a new dance. She slips away from the comforts her mother endured, her mother paid for with her body. She slips away across the tide to her love.

III. "Lovely Joan"

"Lovely Joan"
A fine young man it was indeed
Mounted on his milk-white steed
He rode he rode and he rode all alone
Until he came to lovely Joan

Good morning to you my pretty maid
And Twice good morning sir she said
He tipped her the wink and she rolled her dark eye
Says he to himself I'll be there by and by
Oh don't you think these pooks of hay
A pretty place for us to play?

So come with me me sweet young thing
And I'll give you my golden ring
So he took off his ring of gold
Says me pretty fair miss do this behold
Freely I'll give it for your maidenhead

And her cheeks they blushed like the roses red
Come give that ring into my hand
And I will neither stay nor stand
For your ring is worth much more to me
Than twenty maidenheads said she

And as he made for the pooks of hay
She leapt on his horse and she tore away
He called he called but he called in vain

For Joan she never looked back again
Nor did she think herself quite safe
Until she came to her true love's gate
She'd robbed him of his horse and ring
And she left him to rage in the meadows green

A crimson, gold-speckled maple leaf dances, swirling, through periwinkle early morning. Familiar rain and the spice of a northern New York autumn mingle with eight women's breathing. In the moments between sleep and waking, between three in a line and dancing, legs tingle, summoning energetic movement. Five rest alongside, other dances already soaring, some not yet. Sweet airborne notes.

Three dance in place, unframed driving energy, syncopated. Dancing alive with rhythm and momentum both sustaining dancers and modifying itself to accommodate the dance. Conversations among women, between dancers and musician. Dancing this dance while she dances, while other music takes its own space, to dance in this space without filling in other creative spaces, stilling others' feet.

Three caper fictions into delicious existence, joyfully, deeply, imaginatively. Not all dancers join all dances. Explorers are not welcome to watch, not invited to clear trees, map possibilities, put paradoxical strains neatly into 4/4 time, name exotic and then calculate many dances into complexly straightforward equations. These lives do not dance all pieces; there is no puzzle to be solved.

Three dance lovely Joan, offered a ring of gold for her maidenhead, for her dances. She dances a flexible center, while two circle round. Each moves alone, each moves with the others, circling hands, a flick of the wrist just so. Joy not in power or titillation, but in the love notes of the dance, joy in lovely Joan.

If you read women dancing, eyes liquid in the embers of glowing tongues, perhaps our dances will overlap. Or we'll swim together, icy malachite streams soothing glowing muscles, red-hot energy sizzling under deep swirling waterfalls.

Lovely Joan, enjoying the day, doing her work, wandering alone. "The body is under influence. We have so many words to make it believe that it can, must do this and that, endure that. So many words to increase or diminish its threshold of tolerance" (Brossard 1996, 6). He on his milk white steed, he with his honeyed words and ring of gold. She dances alone and then she leaps and she.

Yes, the body is gregarious. Simple gestures such as to walk, to eat, others more intimate like to cry, laugh, seduce are so much already cultural. . . . Yes, the body is gregarious, but it cares about singularity and intimacy. To take that away from it is to dishonour it.

The body likes to show off but reducing someone to her or his body is to humiliate that person (Brossard 1996, 6).

Lovely Joan takes his ring of gold, whilst he lingers in the hay. Lovely Joan takes his milk white steed. Three dancers close ranks around lovely Joan as she rides away to her love, to her dance, to her freedom. To reduce the body to mute object is to diminish the person, the planet. Three dance lovely Joan, radiant.

IV. "Twa Bonnie Maidens"

"Twa Bonnie Maidens"
There were twa bonnie maidens, and three bonnie maidens,
Cam' owre the Minch, and cam' owre the main,
Wi' the wind for their way and the corry for their hame,
And they're dearly welcome to Skye again.

Come alang, come alang, wi' your boatie and your song,
My ain bonnie maidens, my twa bonnie maids!
For the nicht, it is dark, and the redcoat is gane,
And ye are dearly welcome to Skye again.
There is Flora, my honey, sae dear and sae bonnie,
And ane that's sae tall, and handsome withal.

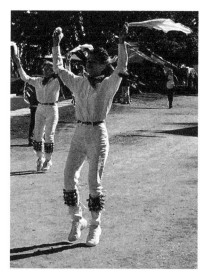

Figure 2.3. Amy Wieber. *B. F. Harridans, Cooperstown, 2004.*

Put the ane for my king and the other for my queen
And they're dearly welcome to Skye again.

Come alang, come alang, w' your boatie and your song,
My ain bonnie maidens, my twa bonnie maids!
For the Lady Macoulain she dwelleth in her lane,
And she'll welcome you dearly to Skye again.
Her arm it is strong, and her petticoat is long,
My ain bonnie maidens, my twa bonnie maidens,
The sea moullit's nest I will watch o'er the main,
And ye are bravely welcome to Skye again.

Come alang, come alang, wi' your boatie and your song,
My ain bonnie maidens, my twa bonnie maids!
And saft sall ye rest where the heather it grows best.
And ye are dearly welcome to Skye again.
There's a wind on the tree, and a ship on the sea,
My ain bonnie maidens, my twa bonnie maids!
Your cradle I'll rock on the lea of the rock,
And ye'll aye be welcome to Skye again.

Come alang, come alang, wi' your boatie and your song,
My ain bonnie maidens, my twa bonnie maids!
Mair sound sall ye sleep as ye rock o'er the deep,
And ye'll aye be welcome to Skye again.

(Note: twa = two; Minch = channel between the Outer and Inner Hebrides; corry = a hollow between mountains.)

There were twa bonnie maidens and three bonnie maidens; there's one who is tall and handsome withall. And two arc out, while two surge forward and two circle back into one long line, expansive and strong. Holding the line, each marks her place until two ease in, two surge forward, two dance away, tracing a new pattern. Playful tune.

Life: dwelling among humans, animals, orange-deep squash flowers, among willowy words. Dancing sardonically, dancing joyfully, this writing, these dances ask: how can one live, live—honoring one's very bones and the stories they hold—in a world where violent death is not only possible but also mundanely common? How to dance so as not to be animated corpses, lulled into lifelessness and deals with the devil?

Two caper slowly, and two continue and two more. There were three bonnie maidens under cover of night. Come along, come along with your boatie and your song. There were two bonnie maidens and bonnie prince Charlie. Six dance a dark night, a night that is long, until the redcoats are gone. Six dance welcome to Skye.

Six dance a story, of disguise. Six dance a story of a man in women's clothing finding a freedom of movement rare for a man pursued, rarer for women, pursued. The writing dances, the writing floats quiet overtones, descants best contemplated in hushed stillness. Sometimes it is meet to pour a libation of dark red wine, silently, for what is held dear and then to close the door as one walks alone in good company, into chilly sunshine, drawing oneself in and never having spoken a word: an act of faith.

There are those modern (and postmodern) travelers, for whom attention to particular embodiment, the turning of the seasons, the minute changes in a place from one day to the next are dross or outside of thought. This traveler moves under the illusion of disembodied superiority in an ignored reliance on others to provide for the needs of the traveler's body, the work and talents and struggles of the producers of food, of shelter, of comfort beyond what the producers themselves often enjoy. The planet groans under the weight of such radical and smug self-indulgence.

"The body has weight, often a moral weight. It can be used as an ultimate argument to protest: to walk naked in a public place, to set oneself on fire in public, to go on a hunger strike. The body never speaks for nothing. If it talks low we can pretend to ignore it, but when it shouts, it becomes terrifying and we must listen" (Brossard 1996, 6). Each dancer has a story, yet to reduce the body to a text is to make it vanish. Six dance, six tempestuous bodies, known intimately to each other after years, after many dances.

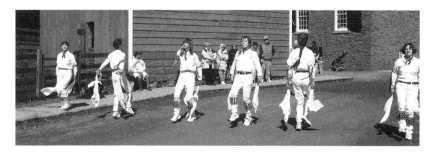

Figure 2.4. Amy Wieber. *B. F. Harridans, Cooperstown, 2004.*

V. The Barrows' House
"Over the Hills and Far Away"

Hark now the drums beat up again
For all true soldier gentlemen
So let us list and march I say
And go over the hills and far away

Chorus:
Over the hills, and o'er the main
To Flanders, Portugal and Spain
Queen Anne commands and we'll obey
And go over the hills and far away

There's twenty shillings on the drum
For him that with us freely comes
'Tis volunteers shall win the day
Over the hills and far away
Chorus
Come gentlemen that have a mind
To serve a queen that's good and kind
Come list and enter in to pay
And go over the hills and far away
Chorus
Prentice Tom may well refuse
To wipe his angry master's shoes
For now he's free to run and play
Over the hills and far away
Chorus
No more from sound of drum retreat
When Marlborough and Galway beat
The French and Spaniards every day
Over the hills and far away.

Mountains expansive, three dancers move with space, kinetic air. She and she and she move with deliberation, close to the ground, fluid. Three dance in formation, three dance futile bravery, three dance to a lone piper's reedy cry.

Writing, words flow from fingertips. The words shape the writer as the dance shapes dancer, bringing themselves onto the page, onto the ground, through the body. When writing fills pages with passionate (or angry), wistful (or winsome), sleepy (or playful) words, the standard bearers, flags flying, have said "poetry." Kind and thoughtful people, imaginative people with golden souls have said "poetry."

Three dance the poetry of the Barrows' Vermont Inn and the dancers who call its mountains home. Three dance the poetry of young men's lives, heeding the call to war, shaping themselves as men, sacrificing and being sacrificed to country, tradition, and promises rarely fulfilled. Three dance a borrowed house, a barrow's house, a mountain house. Three dance, women for whom men claim they go to war. Three dance over the hills and far away. She moves alone, a slow salute. And then she and she, each in turn. And three rotate the triangle to move as one, a sweet refrain—desperate grace.

"Poetry" is sometimes an accusation. Poetry sometimes means writing is not serious, not powerful: a pretty pastime. To separate writing from experience, from emotion, from the body, from beauty is often to reduce writing to a tool, to rob it of its power and its living movement. Instead, to pack the maximum punch, words are to be arranged to erect all the evidence to prove solidly one's point, to win one's argument.

To live in the world mindful of how one's embodiment shapes one's thoughts and how one's thoughts shape how one moves in the world. Thinking from the body, using language that describes one's position in the world with its hurts and pains, injustice and violence, joys and pleasures, is perhaps to use language poetically. I am shy, knowing that my words are often not careful enough, precise enough, mercurial enough, to wear the garland poetry.

Three double step, a slight pull of the arms and hankies back and up so slightly. Three dance to the side, a quick sweep of the wrist. Whether the poetry is literal, pages printed in lines and curves, or figurative, dances wrought or lives lived with care and passion, is not as important as the attention to how one moves in the world and how one reflects on and shapes that moving, to what Audre Lorde calls "the quality of light by which we scrutinize our lives" (1984, 36). This attention is the gift of poetry. Life illuminated in poetic light attends to words and flesh, delight and fear. Lives so animated attend to the tiniest hand unfolding as trees return to green, and to how people move in bodies shaped in the fires of history and the oceans of particular beings.

Six dance, six breath, six move, six live, dancing a window into the work he might have done, the life he might have lived. Six dance for one who went to work at the top of twin mountains, steel and glass, windows on the world and the life he might have lived. Six dance, returning always to earth, for the lives she and she and he and thousands might have lived, two planes and retaliating horror.

A poem can spin dances golden as delicate filigree or as sparse as the oak in winter, adorning language with beauty and pattern, careful, precise, and neat. There can be meditation in the repeated lines of a villanelle, or in a sestina's echoing words. Or the rhyme might return, as in a ballade, telling stories, like dances tracing familiar patterns, the words only being changed. The heart might beat with haiku's spare precision, or well on a moonlit gacela. Words resounding in one person's ear may not ring true against another's tympanum. But lives painted and danced and planted and written in an infinite variety of cultures, in the haunting words, lovely sounds, tortured tones—tongue-caressed, or forsaken—these are the poems of life lived artfully, with all the clumsiness and grace of creation.

> *a rising swan,*
> *surprising on this landscape,*
> *paints your eyelids with fluttering songs,*
> *her wing dipped in opal moonlight.*

Poetic form, too, can bind the tongue, turn haunted lives hollow rather than sending up crooning, keening, aching heartblood on the wings of living words, turn the bones of the quick into a mere skeleton unable to bear the weight of passion. Words shift and change, meanings falling away and new meanings taking shape. Dances change as six dance, tunes shift. Holding words in one's hands, holding dances

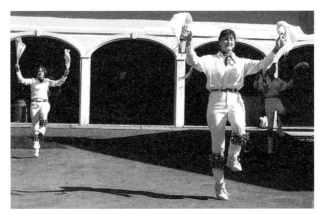

Figure 2.5. Amy Wieber. *B. F. Harridans, Cooperstown, 2004.*

in one's soul, one can sometimes be awed by their power to move, their power to inspire, their power to hurt. Improvisations for the thinking heart, the feeling mind.

Words prepared for battle, standards flying. O'er the hills and o'er the main, through Flanders, Portugal, and Spain. Queen Anne commands and we obey: over the hills and far away. Three dance, and the melody looks back over the fields and fields of dead, a recording angel. Three dance, and writing lives, writing a life without such commands, barrows blooming into kaleidoscopic dances.

Notes

My thanks to the B. F. Harridans, Amy Burtner, kd Davis, Peter Klosky, Michelle Lunt, Jo Malin, Ruth Mitchell, Maria Wackett, and Roberta Wackett for their dances and friendship.

All photographs © by Amy Wieber, September 2004

Works Cited

Brossard, Nicole. 1996. "Only a Body to Measure Reality By: Writing the In-Between." *Journal of Commonwealth Literature* 31:2: 4–17.

Lorde, Audre. 1984. "Poetry Is Not a Luxury." In *Sister Outsider*, ed. Audre Lorde, 36–39. Trumansburg, NY: The Crossing Press.

Smith, Zadie. 2002. *Autograph Man*. New York: Knopf.

3

From Ballet to Boxing

The Evolution of a Female Athlete

Susan Young

It's late July 1979. The rehearsal studio in downtown Toronto is bright and airy, ringed with well-worn gold wood barres and huge windows that look out onto a lush green park. Sunlight spills onto the worn wooden floor where I lie flat on my back, staring up at the ceiling and trying hard to catch my breath. My hair is drenched, and sweat streams steadily down my nose and drips onto the floor, where a small puddle is forming. Only one fan sways back and forth on its stand in the corner; it pushes puffs of hot air around the studio, redolent of fresh sweat, perfume, and wet cotton. Six other dancers are lying on the floor, or leaning exhaustedly against the walls. All of us are panting and sweating profusely. And despite the sweltering heat, all of us are swathed in sweat-soaked layers of plastic and wool, which have been expertly wrapped around and draped over our bodies to protect whatever limbs are currently injured or tight. In my case there's no injury, but I'm trying to get down from 110 to my optimal dance weight of 105 pounds. We're learning a particularly tricky variation from Act II of *Swan Lake* and after company class, partnering class, variations class, and now this rehearsal, it's my fourth hour of hard physical activity today. A faint red stain has seeped through the pink satin of my *pointe* shoe, a reminder that my toe is bleeding again and will have to be rewrapped before I can continue. This elaborate process will take at least ten minutes, since I have to remove the intricate foam padding between each toe, then the thick lamb's wool mummy-wrapped around *that*, and tear off the outer layer of surgical tape binding my toes together. Then I'll have to slather the special homemade dancer's goo composed of antibiotic ointment and anesthetic cream over the torn skin, and repeat the entire process in reverse. Instead, I just stare at my throbbing foot and decide to work through it. Only twenty minutes of rehearsal are left; I can then go and plunge my feet into a bucket of ice.

Ballet was a part of my life from the time my father took me to see my first live performance at age three, a Royal Danish Ballet production of *Copelia*. I finally began studying dance in earnest at the very advanced age of twelve, and from the first class it felt to me as natural as breathing. Einstein once remarked, "Dancers are the athletes of God," and there was certainly something religious about the way I gave myself to dance. Something close to rapture. Three months after my first class I bought a pair of pointe shoes, and after that there was no turning back; ten hours of classes a week and, eventually, acceptance as a corps member in a world-class company. Becoming a dancer initiated my evolution as an athlete, and I began to develop a powerful sense of myself as both female and physical. Even at eighteen, dancing validated my profound belief in a significant and valuable female body ideology unrelated to either of the commonly accepted models for female physicality: reproductive athlete, or competitor for the attention of men. My perspective was only reinforced by joining a community of young women who shared this passion for molding the female body in the interest of creating something other than babies.

Like most adolescent women in Western society, I spent inordinate amounts of time struggling with images of "ideal" female physicality and felt enormous ambivalence about the war this initiated between body and intellect. I was primarily interested in the life of the mind, and I balked at accepting the insipid and ridiculous standards of physical beauty forced on me by the larger culture; at the same time, I was acutely aware of the ease with which those girls who met the standards seemed to move through life. For me the ballet world provided a perfect crucible in which to work through complex issues of female identity and physical Self. Agnes De Mille said, "To dance is to be out of yourself. Larger, more beautiful, more powerful." This was certainly true for me.

The world of professional ballet is delineated by ritual and rules. In its essence, ballet is an art form founded on notions of hierarchy, tradition, conformity, and rigorous self-discipline; every dancer's day begins with a plie and ends with an ache. Most of all, though, ballet is a culture of the body. To a dancer the body is first and always an instrument of artistic expression; one is a dancer first and a woman second. Many of the characteristics that make for a good ballet dancer—musicality, flexibility, an ability to move gracefully—are largely innate; you either have them or you don't. Ballet is also a discipline that demands literal physical restructuring of the body; it glorifies the female body transformed.

As dancers we spent enormous amounts of time working in front of mirrored walls in brightly lit studios where our physiques were on constant public display. Relentless critical self-assessment of the body and a concomitant drive to suppress the physical evidence of female maturation—breasts, hips, fleshy curves—were not only tolerated but professional requirements. In this context, remaining physically prepubescent fed into the practical—that is, biomechanical—requirements of the female dancer. This is because a *ballerina* seeks to present the illusion of weightlessness, of occupying as little space as possible in order to suggest a chaste and an unattainable womanchild. She is a creature of the air, not the earth. Escaping gravity—or at least appearing to do so—is her bread and butter. She is light, graceful, and delicate. She is, as we say in ballet, *pulled up*, all of her weight balanced effortlessly *en pointe*, an area the size of a quarter. In performance, the illusion, both physical and metaphorical, is that she remains perpetually *just out of reach*, but in reality it requires a great deal of sweat and physically punishing effort to create this illusion. It's one of ballet's many inherent paradoxes; the ethereal image of the female dancer belies her tensile strength and toughness.

Like all female dancers I was deeply preoccupied with the geometry created by my body in space, and with the all-important concept of "line." Of course, one of the most efficient ways to create good line is to *be* a line. And here I found myself at a distinct disadvantage, despite my natural ability. I was a textbook mesomorph working in a land where the ectomorph reigns supreme; my tendency was, and is, toward muscularity and strength. My advanced variations teacher, Freda Crisp, peering in despair over the rims of her bifocals at my well-muscled thighs, once declared, "Darling girl, you just have to face it: you're a panther, not a swan." The comment was devastating; I wanted to be a swan, not a panther. However, ruthless critique is part of ballet life, and her observation rang true despite its sting. I was indeed surrounded by ghostly pale swans, lithe and long-limbed sylphs with no breasts, no body fat, impossibly long legs and arms, and tiny heads.

Nonetheless, inasmuch as I was often self-conscious and miserable about my shortcomings as a ballerina, it was in the harsh light of ballet's unrelenting demand for physical honesty that I learned to assess my strengths as a dancer and to compensate for the liabilities. I was unusually flexible (even by ballet standards), quick, light, and powerful (invariably, I was assigned variations designated *con brio*) and had a great deal of what dancers call *ballon*, the ability to jump easily and high. I also had perfect ballet feet; slender with very high arches and sheered-across toes (in ballet lexicon this is known rather unprettily as *peasant toes*) that adapted easily to *pointe* work. And my low center of gravity allowed me to balance for long periods of time *en pointe*, a sort of balletic circus trick. Another useful talent was my ability to see choreography just once—even long sequences of steps—and immediately commit it to muscle memory.

In actuality I wasn't *that* physically different from the other girls in the company; in fact, at 5'4" and barely over 100 pounds I was often dangerously underweight. But unlike many of the other girls, it was hard work for me to maintain a classical dancer's physique. However, we all had methods for subduing our developing women's bodies. Some girls smoked. Others took amphetamines, were bulimic, or slept in their plastic warm-ups for a few days before every company weigh-in. Then there was bee pollen, royal jelly, exotic vitamin supplements, and special herbal teas. I resorted to borderline anorexia as my weapon of choice. During one notorious six-week period I ate nothing but air-popped popcorn, vitamins, stewed tomatoes, canned mushrooms, coffee, and diet cola. The result of this ridiculous regimen was extreme fatigue and nosebleeds, but I was finally reed thin. The panther had transformed herself into a very pale, very tired swan.

Despite being a "panther in swan's clothing," I was happy overall as a dancer. More than happy. Ecstatic. It is impossible for anyone other than another dancer to understand the joy of those elusive, perfect moments when your body, the music, your emotions, and the power of brilliant choreography come together in such a way that self and art become indistinguishable. For me, the continual self-discipline and punishing physical rigor were justified in those breathtaking, transcendent moments on stage. Unlike the messy and complex world of female adolescence, this was a world where I was in control, at least of my body; a world where things were ordered and disciplined and beautiful.

There was tremendous warmth and camaraderie among the female dancers in the company. We were united not only by the extraordinary physical demands of our profession but also because we were members of a small, elite community with a unique skill set. And despite the melodrama of ballet movies such as *The Turn-*

ing Point and *Center Stage*, where female dancers are at each other's throats in a vicious rivalry for lead roles, in real life that kind of dynamic is rare. I never saw it. In fact, my experience taught me valuable lessons about mentorship and collaboration among women. In a professional company, dancers are too interdependent to waste time on petty jealousies and useless competition. In fact, many of the other female dancers mentored me and were unfailingly generous in sharing their expertise—helping me learn complex variations, giving me advice about everything from how to heal injuries, apply stage makeup, break in toe shoes (repeated slamming in a door jamb works best), and disguise my physical limitations as a dancer, and telling me how best to work with demanding choreographers.

Injury and age are the enemies of every dancer and are the reasons dance careers tend to be short. On average, a professional dancer's career spans seven to ten years. When I was twenty-one, my short career in dance came to an abrupt end with a serious knee injury, the result of falling out of an overhead lift I was practicing with an inexperienced partner. At the time I was learning a beautiful variation set to the *romanza larghetto* section of Chopin's exquisite Piano Concerto No. 1 in E Minor. It's still my favorite piece of classical music, and it still brings me to tears whenever I hear it. Although it seemed I'd never get past the pain and disappointment of having to give up ballet, at twenty-one both the mind and the body are resilient. I left classical dance with a powerful foundation of physical and psychological tools, the most valuable being a profound love of movement. So much of what I did and learned as a dancer set the context for my subsequent life as an athlete.

Not long ago I came across a photo taken during what my brother calls the "tutu era." The pale young woman gazing out at the camera looks serene, with huge green eyes perched above angular cheekbones, blonde hair pulled back in a perfect ballet bun encircled by a shimmering cascade of rhinestones, with not a single hair out of place. Her collarbone juts sharply above the strapless neckline of her "Snowflake" costume, and a faint smile drifts across her lips; she looks ethereal and vaguely haunted. In one sense I don't recognize her as myself. Looking at that photo today, one thing is certain: I may have been happy when it was taken, but I was not yet a physically empowered woman.

I became a figure skater by accident. While I had always been passionate about ballet, I had never been remotely interested in figure skating. In fact, although my parents had taken me to see live ice shows and I'd enjoyed them as a spectator, I always wondered what would possess anyone in her right mind to spend so much time training in a cold arena, wear those dumb costumes, and freeze her keister off. Also, compared to the aesthetic ideal I'd internalized as a ballet dancer, skaters were bulky and overly muscular. But the year I turned thirty, I wound up in Manhattan's *Skyrink* taking an adult beginner skating class, having reluctantly tagged along to keep a friend company.

Through my teens and twenties dance had been my refuge; even after moving to New York and beginning doctoral studies, I took dance classes several times a week. There were always the familiar sights, sounds, and smells: big mirrored walls, the tinny sound of the live piano, the humid hothouse air of a well-used studio, and the chalky smell of rosin mixed with the scents of fresh sweat and perfumed body talc. Taking class, with all of its rituals, felt like going home after a long and tiring journey. It was also a way to stay in peak condition and offset the stresses of teaching, studying, and adjusting to life in Manhattan. But by the time I found myself alongside a dozen other adults, all awkwardly lurching around the rink in cheap blue rental skates, I'd grown tired of ballet classes. I didn't need the familiarity of daily *pliés* anymore, or the self-assurance derived from knocking off tricky variations from *La Bayadere*. I still loved dance; I just didn't want to *do* it anymore. I'd outgrown ballet, mentally and physically. My body ideology had evolved.

The first time I stepped gingerly onto that huge milky sheet of ice, it felt like home. Suddenly I could move freely, powerfully, with very little effort. Reader, I was hooked! Every week I trudged across Manhattan to *Skyrink* after a full day at the college where I had secured a full-time teaching job. Every week I loved skating more and more and would stay later and later after the lesson to practice what I'd learned from the chaotic public skating sessions. Every lesson left me eager and impatient for the following week's class. I started coming two extra times a week just to practice. As an ex-dancer I understood the necessity of learning fundamental concepts before attempting showy tricks and bravura maneuvers, and knew that talent is no hedge against solid technique. So I spent many frustrating hours mastering basic skating edgework: three-turns, brackets, front and back crossovers, Choctaws and Mohawks. (And no, I have no idea why so many skating steps are named after Native American tribes, since I have yet to see a Native American figure skater.) Before a skater jumps or spins at anything other than the most rudimentary level, these movements must become so organic to her physical vocabulary that the difference between walking on the ground and moving on ice is virtually indistinguishable.

There's no doubt that my ballet experience was an enormous advantage—both physical and psychological—in learning to skate. Ballet had instilled a strong sense of physical self-discipline, the patience to persevere through the often-frustrating process of learning new and difficult skills, a high degree of knowledge about my body's capabilities and limitations, and, of course, balance, rhythm, and flexibility. And I could tolerate considerable pain. But there were many realities of the sport that dance had not prepared me for, such as taking frequent hard falls on ice or making abrupt changes of direction at high rates of speed (the learning curve for this skill is particularly steep, often resulting in a singularly ungraceful fall known among skaters as a "face-plant"). In the process of learning complex spin combinations and multirevolution jumps, I suffered injuries foreign to ballet dancers: a cracked ankle bone, a black eye, and a badly swollen knee on a double Lutz attempt (the result of stupidly refusing to use a training harness), a concussion when I fell backwards out of a layback spin, and several deep cuts (one obtained when I somehow managed to skate over my own finger). Until I mastered falling out of jumps, there frequently were bruises as big as dinner plates all over my thighs, back, and butt. Anyone who debates whether figure skating is an art or a sport obviously doesn't skate.

The optimal body for ladies figure skating has a low center of gravity, long arms for increased balance, a long torso for spinal flexibility (important in camel and layback spins), fast-twitch muscles, and a mesomorphic build that lend power, speed, and elevation to jumps, fast rotational momentum to spins, and quickness and precision to footwork. It had taken me thirty years to find it, but I'd finally stumbled onto a sport for which I had the right body. Elite female figure skaters are lean but far more muscular than ballet dancers, especially in the lower body. Muscle begets muscle, and protecting muscle mass while maintaining a lean—not thin—physique is the goal of every competitive female figure skater.

Another aspect I found appealing was the inherent gender equity of the sport. Both males and females are subject to the same laws of physics that govern the process of learning figure skating. A skater—male or female—must understand the mechanical laws that govern rotational momentum, or know that the precise optimal angle for a landing leg coming out of a jump, relative to the ice surface, is 108 degrees. None of this is gender-dependent. The playing field—as slippery as it is—is generally level in terms of gender. Spin for spin and jump for jump, male and female skaters go through the same training process, take the same falls, and receive the same coaching instruction. Acquiring these complex skills is more a matter of finesse than muscular force. In fact, one of the most negative comments a coach makes to a skater learning multirevolution jumps is that she or he "muscled" the jump.

After eight weeks of group classes, my instructor pulled me aside and suggested I switch to private coaching, explaining that although costly, private instruction would benefit me more than group classes if I wanted to pursue skating as a serious hobby. In figure skating there is an intensely personal element of collaboration between coach and athlete, and the skater has to trust a coach enough to place her physical welfare in his or her hands, so two weeks later I showed up for my first lesson with Doug Webster, a former USFSA national competitor. I watched him skate in a professional freestyle session and was blown away by his aggressive, powerful style. He took absolute command of the ice, executing huge, dazzling jumps that left him momentarily suspended in air, and he spun so quickly it made me dizzy just watching him. Most importantly, there was a feline, feral quality to his skating that called out my own inner "panther." He appropriated space in a wild, abandoned way that is only possible in an athlete who has complete mastery over his medium. Even as a thirty-year-old—and in skating terms, positively geriatric—athlete, I wanted more than anything in the world to experience that quality of movement.

At our initial lesson he told me to skate around for a few minutes, and then he demonstrated some simple steps and asked me to mimic them to get a sense of my skating ability. He asked about my goals as a skater; I already knew. Having achieved an elite level of proficiency in one physical realm, I was realistic about my options in this one. I wanted to learn to jump, spin, and skate with some semblance of mastery and confidence, but I wasn't interested in serious competitive skating, even in the adult category. He countered with some cold, hard truths about the limits of what I could hope to achieve as an adult beginner. But as a dancer I was no stranger to harsh truths. He said double jumps were possible, and he felt I could learn them with hard work and a considerable commitment of time. Triple jumps were out of the question; I'd started about twenty years too late. He felt I had good ability for advanced spinning, and that learning complex footwork was simply a matter of how much time, money, and tedious repetition I was willing to invest. And so, after the first hour of what turned out to be an eight-year coaching relationship, I went home sore and humbled but determined to excel in this new sport.

As a dancer I had never moved my body with the kind of unbridled aggressive power that skating demands, because ballet is largely about control and restraint, even when it appears to suggest abandonment; that too is an illusion. In skating there is little room for illusions, because the sport demands frank athleticism, regardless of the amount of sequins, feathers, or beaded chiffon the skater wears in performance. Those are the props used to foster the impression that it's easy to barrel down a sheet of ice at twenty miles an hour on a steel blade a quarter of an inch thick, launch oneself into the air, rotate two or more times in less than a second, and return safely to earth—smiling—all the while balanced on that same quarter inch of steel. But before the elaborate costumes and choreography, a skater first has to master complex skills that require intelligence, raw courage, and a lot of physical self-confidence. Forceful, decisive movement is important in skating, because if the skater hesitates going into a jump, or zones out entering a spin combination, well, let's just say that nothing good will come of it. To excel at higher-level skills such as double jumps or combination spins requires either trying 100 percent or not at all; there's no "sort of" trying in freestyle skating. As Doug liked to say, "Go hard, or go home."

I also discovered that the everyday reality of a serious figure skater requires solitary, self-driven commitment to the sport that has nothing to do with sparkling costumes, spotlights, or applause. Once I began to pursue skating as a serious avocation, I was plunged into a world of early morning "patch" sessions, where the dimly lit rink is divided into several "patches" of ice on which skaters silently practice edgework; these are the elaborate and difficult "figures" for which the sport is named. Then there were ice dancing lessons, instruction in "moves in the field," where skaters practice complex sequences of steps strung together over the entire ice surface, and, of course, private freestyle lessons to learn jumps and spins. The time and expense are considerable. My custom-made boots and blades cost $700, while ice time and coaching fees added up to about $15,000 a year. A serious *competitive* skater preparing to make skating her profession spends at least $75,000 a year on training, equipment, costumes, choreographers, music arrangers, competition and testing fees, and travel. And the time demands are equally rigorous; in the first five years of training, I got up at 4 a.m. three times a week to skate two or three hours before putting in a full day of teaching and meetings. Often I would return to the rink after work for another hour of practice.

A year after I began private lessons I earned the right to skate in advanced freestyle sessions, where I frequently shared the ice with the best skaters in the sport; world and Olympic champions such as Brian Boitano, Scott Hamilton, Michelle Kwan, Tara Lipinski, Oksana Baiul, and Katerina Witt. Russian ice dancers tore around at speeds so fast my hair blew back when they passed me. When Doug took me into my first pro session it was like being launched into a particle accelerator. I remember turning to him and saying, "This may not be the best session for me to start on." He gave me a gentle shove and said, "Get out there. Figure it out." Terrified, I took my first shaky step onto the ice and tentatively moved into the chaotic slipstream of high-level figure skating. Pro sessions are intimidating; each skater works in a self-contained bubble of concentration while simultaneously having to monitor the whereabouts of fifteen other skaters on the ice, all moving at very high rates of speed, performing difficult, and often dangerous, maneuvers, and all going in different directions. The elite female skaters in the pro sessions were particularly compelling to me because they provided the best possible role models both in their technical excellence and in establishing a work ethic on the ice. These women taught me how to really "work" the sessions, and they frequently and generously took time out of their own workouts to offer suggestions, to share insider tips, or to demonstrate when they saw me struggling again and again to master a jump or spin.

Never one to do anything by halves, I started taking USFSA tests in three disciplines: figures, freestyle, and ice dancing. Testing was easy for me, not because skating was simple, but because I knew how to perform, understood the need to rehearse my choreography until it was perfect, and never took criticism from the judges personally. My pile of test certificates grew steadily; every month I'd go out there alone on that vast sheet of ice and let the USFSA judges—the same ones who judge world and Olympic competitors—determine whether or not I met the standards of the sport. Usually I passed, but sometimes I failed, and in doing so I learned not just about my shortcomings as an athlete but also about the subjective element inherent in figure skating. In one instance a judge failed me on three separate occasions because she didn't like the way I skated one of the steps in a thirty-five-step dance sequence.

I competed twice as a skater at the master's intermediate level and hated it both times, even though I won. I'd come to know several of the women against whom I was competing and liked them immensely; I felt no pleasure in their slips or falls. We all trained together and had in fact often helped each other with tricky footwork, or a difficult jump, or centering a spin. Skating is a sport where competition results in only one winner, and it takes only one tiny mistake, one wrongly placed foot or missed landing on a jump that you've nailed hundreds of times in practice, to lose. It became very clear that I didn't have the necessary "killer instinct" when I found myself at a competition waiting to perform my program and the competitor ahead of me—a woman with whom I'd shared many practice sessions—sped down-ice into a particularly challenging jump combination. I found myself mentally running through the maneuver with her, willing her to make the jump successfully. She did, and I felt relief. That's when I knew for sure I didn't have a competitor's temperament; I loved performing, but I just didn't see the point of competing.

Unlike ballet, skating is at its heart a solitary sport. You may compete against other women or perform in ensemble numbers if you're in an ice show, but the vast majority of time is spent practicing and performing alone, whether on a test, in a competition, or as a featured performer in a show. There is also a distinctly exhibitionistic aspect to the sport; you have to, somewhere deep in your soul, *like* showing off. And you have to want to win badly enough to mentally detach yourself from the losses that your win will mean for your competitors, whether they're off-ice friends or not. In the minds of Olympic and world competitors, it's not personal; it's their job to win. As Doug once told me before a competition: "Just get on, do your job, and get off." Despite my own indifference to the competitive aspects of the sport, skating taught me a lot about the nature of *healthy* competition. I learned that it's possible to compete vigorously in a way that is impersonal but simultaneously respects the hard work and skill of other women. I also realized that in figure skating, winning is often just a matter of having a lucky day. Two skaters may be equally matched in ability and skills, but an unexpected case of nerves, failure to get enough sleep the night before, or the distraction of a loose skate lace can determine who wins.

My relationships with other female skaters, on both professional and recreational levels, have been the most rewarding legacy of my involvement with the sport. Over the years I forged strong and lasting friendships with several women who came to the sport like I did, as adults. We were women of different races, professions, sexualities, nationalities, and ages, but we formed a close-knit community through our passion for skating. Dubbing ourselves the Rink Ratz, we met at least once a week for dinner to share the sordid stories of our (mis)adventures on the ice, brag about our triumphs as adult athletes, and bemoan our painful humiliations. All of the women I met when

I began skating have remained close friends for over fifteen years. Although most of the Rink Ratz have quit the sport, a few of us have stayed the course, but all of us have been profoundly transformed by its beauty and challenges.

So how did figure skating advance my evolution as a feminist athlete? Becoming a skater in my thirties coincided with a sea change in my ideas about what constitutes physical beauty in women in general, and me in particular. For one thing, I permanently dropped the word "dieting" from my vocabulary and haven't used it, or done it, since. Where dysfunctional eating habits in the ballet world were not only rarely questioned but in fact obliquely encouraged, anorexia and bulimia among skaters were, and are, universally greeted with disapproval. Moreover, my contact with elite women in the sport, watching them practice and perform at close range, reinforced for me the importance of feeding my muscles well and nurturing their strength. Every time I spent one thrilling airborne instant at the top of a double flip, I thanked my muscular thighs for getting me up there. I loved the new bulk and definition of my skater's legs. When Doug told me approvingly that my jumps were powerful, and "solid," I remembered how pejorative those words would have been in my ballet life, how they would have tormented me. The vocabulary of skating reshaped my aesthetic sense of female physicality. Where the body ideology of classical ballet had driven me—at great physical and emotional expense—to disguise my natural physique in an outwardly fragile and ethereal appearance, skating liberated me with its emphasis on power, speed, grace, and physical courage.

An unexpected bonus of my passion for skating came in the form of numerous opportunities to experience the lifestyle of a working professional. I was recruited to do skating exhibitions, experimental ice dance performances, and to skate at charity events under the auspices of Ice Theatre of New York. I took advanced workshops with JoJo Starbuck, the Olympic pair skater whose grace, kindness, and mentorship helped me polish my on-ice performance skills (skating fast on a dark sheet of ice under the blinding glare of moving spotlights is a very long way from doing *Swan Lake*). I skated in promotional events at Rockefeller Center for AOL and the Canadian embassy. I did TV spots, was featured in a spread on adult skating in the *New York Post*, and did several fashion shows on ice. I even skated a gig as a giant Raggedy Andy doll in a promotional event at the South Street Seaport in Manhattan.

Although I skate infrequently these days, I know I'll return to ice dancing at some point. But there's a new athletic love in my life (more about that shortly). The wonderful thing is that skating is a sport I'll be able to return to for the rest of my life; at age seventy-five I probably won't be jumping or spinning, but I will certainly be able to put on those hard white boots with their glinting Sheffield steel blades, inhale the unmistakable scent of cold rink air, and glide onto the mist-covered ice of an early morning Seniors Session.

I'm not a believer in using physical aggression for any reason other than to defend one's life. Prior to taking up boxing, the most physically aggressive thing I'd ever done was dump a plate of hot linguine into the lap of a blind date who suggested that I'd look a lot better if I got breast implants. So it surprised me that I loved boxing the first time I threw a punch. Having joined a neighborhood gym two years ago, I was going several times a week but was becoming bored with the monotony of cardio training and the light weight routine I'd picked up from various fitness magazines. That's when I met Felicia. I'd already decided I wanted a female trainer, but she impressed me in several respects. Most importantly, she had a college degree in kinesiology and was articulate and knowledgeable about human anatomy. She was also a Marine drill sergeant. But what sealed the deal was when she asked me at our first workout session what my fitness goals were, and before I could answer she told me that if my goal was to be skinny, I shouldn't waste my time, because she was not the trainer for me. I replied that I had no interest in being a size zero—I'd "been there, done that"—but wanted to develop more muscle, especially in the upper body. At forty-three, with three decades of athletic achievement behind me, I was no longer haunted by the specter of ballet-body perfection, and I had absolutely no interest in meeting anybody's image standards except my own. Now I wanted to pare down my athleticism to its elemental core. No sequins, no chiffon, no music, no sylphlike illusions.

After six months of hard-core gym training with Felicia I knew how to use every single machine in the gym and spent two hours a week in the weight room, where I was usually the only woman. The training ethic acquired from both ballet and skating carried over into my work with Felicia: discipline, perseverance, love of movement, tolerance for pain and frustration, and an instinctive kinesthetic sense. I learned about dropsets, negative reps, pyramid sets, and supersets. Ironically, although I was older when I started weight training, I felt stronger and less fatigued by these hard-core workouts than I had felt when I was a dancer. The notion that a woman could become stronger and more physically fit even as she aged lodged itself in my mind, and the proof was in the mirror. With Felicia's stringent guidance, I began to see visible changes in my body; I became more muscular, a full-flowering mesomorph with well-defined biceps and broadened shoulders. My abs, which had always been well defined and flat, began to feel tighter, even as a little layer of premenopausal fat started to sneak across my midsection. On the other hand, I suddenly had pecs. Big ones.

But the real turning point came when I showed up to train one day and Felicia pulled out a battered pair of red boxing gloves from her gym bag. "I think you should try boxing," she said. I burst into laughter. "I'm a dancer, a skater. Not a boxer," I replied, and then executed an off-ice axel to punctuate my point. Felicia stared back at me impassively. "I think you'll be good at this," she said. "You have the right build and you're strong." "Really?" I replied, laughing. "Is there a geriatric boxing club? Perhaps a *Golden Years* Golden Gloves?" But even as I joked, that old familiar excitement kicked in, the irresistible curiosity guaranteed to lure an athlete to a new, unconquered sport. Felicia persisted. "Just try an hour of drills, and if you hate it, we won't do it again." This seemed reasonable, so I pulled on the big bulky training gloves and began boxing.

Another decade, another sport. I was the only woman boxing at the gym, and the other women watched me; some looked confused, some looked anxious. Boxing, I realized, is a sport so definitively associated with masculinity that the sight of a woman throwing punches and liking it is visibly disturbing to many people, both male and female. Women think it's unnatural and somehow unfemale, and men feel an uneasy sense of encroachment. A woman who boxes crosses some invisible gender line of athletic propriety. And so I immersed myself in a new kind of training, one devoid of the gender-based, apologist trappings afforded by glittering costumes, sylphlike slenderness, and beautiful music. Boxing and weight training derive from elemental physicality. Felicia taught me how to throw punch combinations in rapid-fire succession, to duck and weave, to dance lightly on my feet like a boxer, *not*—she often emphasized—like a ballerina. Oddly enough, there are some surprising correlations between dance, skating, and boxing. Far from being the brutal and senselessly violent sport I had always thought it to be, boxing requires power and fast reflexes (like skating), a great sense of timing, flexibility, and choreography (like ballet) and physical confidence, coupled with aggression (skating, again). Boxing, I now know from experience, is inarguably a skill sport.

What's more, few athletic endeavors can reshape the entire body like boxing can, primarily because of the rigorous drills that form the underpinning of a boxer's conditioning regimen. Felicia had me doing what seemed like endless sets of regular and decline push-ups on my knuckles while wearing my gloves, hundreds upon hundreds of crunches, and, of course, long stretches of punching sequences that whipped my upper body into shape like nothing I'd experienced before. New words entered my lexicon: jab, cross, uppercut, and hook. And I discovered why boxing rounds are short; three minutes of continuous punching, bobbing, and weaving feels like an eternity and leaves me gasping for air. With every week of boxing drills I feel more and more physically empowered; bigger and stronger, but no less feminine than when I was a pale and lovely cygnet dancing in *Swan Lake*. Unlike ballet, however, boxing demands the athlete's physical dominance over space and assumes that the body commands the space it occupies rather than simply moving within it. In learning how to box, I've arrived at a place where the relevance of gender, societal constructs about the physical female body, and even age, is secondary to the importance of athletic skill.

The real extent of my evolution from ballet dancer to fledgling boxer was brought home to me one sweltering summer day last July as I made my way home from work. Passing through a subway turnstile in Manhattan, a man coming through in the opposite direction suddenly reached out and grabbed my breast. My response was instantaneous and reflexive; I clocked him with a hard left hook to the side of his head. He staggered backwards, nearly falling flat on his butt, cursing savagely the whole time. Three large men nearby witnessed what happened and were on their way over to help me when I landed the blow. They were nearly as shocked as I was. My heart pounded furiously, and I felt adrenaline flood my body, but I wasn't afraid. My knuckles hurt for the rest of the day; nevertheless, the action came from a place of deep strength and empowerment, a place where I had been trained to respond decisively. Now, we can argue all day about the advisability of doing what I did. But the cold, hard truth of the matter is that I wasn't a sylph anymore, and my response wasn't that of a ballet heroine: suicide, lapsing into suspended animation, or transforming into a bird. At age forty-five, I'd traveled several decades and a million miles from the rail-thin, luminous sixteen-year-old girl who was eager to dance herself into exhaustion for the sake of high art.

These days I go to the gym four times a week and spend an hour and a half there. Sometimes there are a couple of women in the weight room; many times I'm the only one. But it feels comfortable to be there and even better when other women show up. We work together in silence, side by side, occasionally asking each other for

spotting on a set of bench presses, or for help with lifting on negative reps.

I've danced, skated, and boxed my way to understanding
that escape from body image tyranny is not a matter of revelation
but evolution. A crucial factor in this process for me has been the
presence and encouragement of other women—seasoned ballerinas,
ice-dancing coaches, personal trainers, and other female athletes,
professional and amateur alike—who presented me with dazzling
models of athleticism and strength outside the limiting definitions
under which I struggled as an adolescent. In *Survival of the Prettiest*
Nancy Etcoff writes about the negative impact of women's criticism of
each other's bodies: "Why is there so much self-denigration and envy?
Because every woman somehow finds herself, without her consent,
entered into a beauty contest with every other woman. No matter
how irrelevant to her goals, how inappropriate to her talents and
endowments, or how ridiculous the comparison, women are always
compared to one another and found wanting" (Etcoff 2000, 68). I've
seen and experienced this kind of intragender nastiness all too often,
but rarely among female athletes, since the competitiveness—however
ferocious—is usually channeled into athletic expression. Love of dance
and sport has brought me into contact with so many athletically
talented women with whom I've forged strong connections based
on mutual reinforcement, mentorship, and respect. Over time, this
has freed me from the corrosive and competitive judgment process
that many of us reflexively apply to each other, a process that runs
counter to any notion of universal female empowerment. Ironically,
the more hard core my training becomes, the easier it is to finally
and completely shed the unhealthy and woman-negative images of
female physicality foisted onto all of us from the time we're born
until the day we fall—either skinny and starving, or "overweight"
and self-loathing—into the grave.

Recently I watched an *Animal Planet* documentary about the big
cats; there was footage of lions, cheetahs, and panthers, their glorious bodies monuments of muscle and sinew, racing after prey on
the veldts of Africa or launching themselves into the jungle trees of
South America with breathtaking power and grace. I thought about
my ballet teacher, Freda Crisp, and the disappointed tone in her voice
when she told me I'd never be a swan, that I was too much like a
panther. Thirty years later, I'm happy to say that she was absolutely
right. I'm not a swan; I *am* a panther. A forty-five-year-old panther
with a nasty left hook.

Works Cited

Etcoff, Nancy. 2000. *Survival of the Prettiest: The Science of Beauty*. New York: Anchor Books.

Garafola, Lynn, ed. 1997. *Rethinking the Sylph: New Perspectives on the Romantic Ballet*. Middletown, CT: Wesleyan University Press.

4

The Women's Dance

Virginia Corrie-Cozart

"The Women's Dance"

After the best man's speech
and the Episcopal formalities,
the musicians declared a ladies' dance.

We stepped to the edges
in our high heels and silks,
watched our toes test the new rhythm.

Lightened by music,
we formed a circle around the bride,
who was made bold by the ring.

She tucked back her veil,
led with her hips
and swung back her head,

the Turkish dancer
who tells the courtship story,
playful and sinuous,
foretells childbirth with undulations.

We connected arm across shoulder,
improvising rapturous Aphrodite.

For Hera, fierce protector of wives,
we shared steps as we recalled them,
precise grapevine to the left, the right.

Our circle became a line
that coiled around a druid in white satin,
our scalds and bruises acknowledged
in significant ellipses.

Advised which ones could be healed,
which were beyond the help
of our touches and potions.

We rushed our seed-pearl center
with joined hands,
a village toast to the queen,
arms high, a whoop at the end.

Our wave receded like outgoing salt water,
then poured in again.

Exultation for the power of oceans.
We showed each other the calluses
of our gestures:
smoothing of skirts over laps,
spreading of linens on beds,
stroking of countless foreheads.

We shared the pain
we enter into gladly.

The music stopped,
our muscles quivering.

Did the young groom notice,
the old husbands know
how we walked back proudly,
as women,
to the banquet tables,
the tables of men?

Part 2

■

The Gym, Weight Room, Studio, and Pool

5

You Spin Me Right Round, Baby

Resistance, Potential, and
Feminist Pedagogy in Indoor Cycling

Kristine Newhall

I could say I go to the gym to keep fit, reduce stress, become stronger, and stay flexible and agile—and I would not be lying. But these reasons constitute only part of my motivation; it is only part of what gets me out of bed before 6 a.m. to lift weights or steers the car toward the gym after a long day. Because like the majority of other women in the gym, I started going to lose weight. And losing weight is still part of the reason I work out—whether or not I admit that to myself every time I walk through those doors.

Since my early twenties, when I began a regular workout routine, all of the reasons I just listed have accumulated, and their importance grows as I continue to go to the gym. But the process of coming to value things such as stress reduction and building strength over weight loss is a perpetual one that requires constant negotiation. This is, in part, due to the atmosphere in the gym. I wish that the gym could be a safe and supportive space with a discernible community of members, owners, managers, and instructors that encourages all types of people to engage in and succeed at physical fitness and the creation of a healthy lifestyle. I would like it to be a community that stresses participation and sets goals that contribute to a healthy lifestyle. But that has not been my experience. Whenever I enter the gym—any gym I have ever belonged to—a ticker tape of defensive thoughts, directed at real and imaginary persons, runs across my mind: *yes, I can press that weight; no, I am not almost done; and yes, I was actually planning on using that barbell.* I sound bitter, irritated, bordering on bitchy even. And while I don't actually say these things, I do not want to be mired down by these feelings in a space that should be encouraging positive thoughts. But when I walk into a gym to start my workout, I am acutely aware that I have entered—if not an outright misogynist—then certainly a patriarchal space, often infused with a paradoxical homophobic/homoerotic aura. Despite encountering an *emphasis* on a friendly and noncompetitive space, my observations suggest that this is not enough to counter the highly gendered[1] atmosphere that permeates.

This chapter serves as an entry point into a larger ethnographic study of the gym in which I examine the gendered atmosphere of the space and seek to better understand the power dynamics exerted by and on members—specifically female members—and how we negotiate the often conflicting messages present in the space of the gym. My conception of the space and these dynamics is informed by Bourdieu's concept of field: a discernible, ordered space that has a history that is recognizable to its participants. Bourdieu explicitly stated that sport itself is a field—comprised of many subfields—but here I present the gym as its own field that contains a number of subfields (1984, 208–209). In contrast to institutional and recreational sport, the gym is situated in a complex intersection of public and private space, oftentimes serving as a transition or an intermediary point between what we delineate as the boundary between home and work/public life. We fit the gym into our daily lives often in a transitional moment of the day. Perhaps in the morning we leave home, go to the gym, and go to work. Or, at the end of the day, it is work, gym, home. The clothes we wear are neither work clothes nor casual. We are not performing in the same way (though we certainly are performing!) in the gym as we do at work or at home. Working out is private leisure time spent in a public space. But it is just this complexity that draws me to investigate the space that has become integral to my daily life.

So I begin this study with an account of my own participation in "gym culture," focusing on one of the activities that has helped me negotiate my own place in the gym: indoor cycling. My work here is informed by feminist scholars of sport, including Theberge, Haravon Collins, and, later, Markula, who have highlighted women's participation in aerobics as both limiting and liberating. Theberge writes that the American fitness boom of the 1980s targeted women who were participating in greater numbers in activities that encouraged strength building and endurance training. Simultaneously, activities such as dance aerobics and Jazzercise gained popularity. But these workouts endeavored to sexualize women rather than to make them more powerful. Theberge argues that their ubiquity caused a "femininization of the fitness movement," the result of which was "not the liberation of women in sport, but their continued oppression though the sexualization of physical activity" (1987, 389).

In her study of women in dance aerobics, Haravon Collins's informants spoke of the oppressive aspects of aerobics, such as the revealing attire, instructors' comments about food and diet, and the male gaze present in the gym (2002, 93–94). The juxtaposition of empowerment and oppression in aerobics presents a contradiction that the author acknowledges. But she argues that women can use the empowering practices imbedded in aerobic dance to make sense of the contradictions, even if they cannot be overcome (106).

Paradoxical situations such as this one complicate our understanding of an empowerment rhetoric that claims physical activity as the key to overcoming low self-esteem, poor body image, and general feelings of powerlessness in and outside the gym. Discussing the empowerment potential in spaces such as the gym or the aerobics classroom forces us to contend with conflicting ideologies about exercise, fitness, and healthy lifestyles. Indoor cycling shares many of the same problems with dance aerobics. Because it occurs within the space of the gym and thus has been incorporated into the larger fitness industry, indoor cycling also sends—often through the instructors themselves—problematic messages about body image and the goals of exercise that limit women's access to physical and emotional self-improvement, overall health, and empowerment. But there are also significant differences between indoor cycling and aerobics that make it a potentially empowering activity for women. I have used it to negotiate my own conflicts over my presence in the gym both as a participant and as an instructor.

Because indoor cycling is a relatively new gym activity (as compared to other forms of aerobics), little research focuses on its practice or its distinction from other forms of group exercise. The activity merits its own consideration, especially given its hybrid nature. Indoor cycling is, in some ways, outdoor cycling adapted for consumption by cyclists and gym goers alike. Indoor cycling can simulate an outdoor training ride, or it can be an intense aerobic and anaerobic workout done on a stationary bike.

Indoor cycling entered gyms in the 1990s after the initial step aerobics craze. And fitness giant Reebok[2] had a hand in this phenomenon too, though many other companies manufacture bikes and have patented their own indoor cycling programs. It is a fairly simple concept: a room full of stationary bikes, with instructors who lead participants through various drills, which create both a cardio and strength workout, all set to music. It appeals to a wider demographic than traditional aerobics classes because of the mix of a cardio and strength workout and because it is not marked as "feminine" in the same ways traditional aerobics programs have been. Outdoor cycling enthusiasts, including men, who comprise the majority of professional and amateur cyclists, can participate in indoor cycling to stay in shape during the off season. It also presents a change to the monotony of traditional cardio workouts on elliptical trainers, stair-steppers, and treadmills. And because it has not been feminized and sexualized in the same way that step aerobics or Jazzercise has, it is, in theory, more inclusive of a diverse group of people.

This last aspect was what finally, several years after the craze hit my gym, got me into a class. I was only mildly impressed after my first experience. But I gave my sore butt a week to recover and then gave it a second chance. Not long after, I went out and bought cycling shoes (so I could clip into the pedals) and a special seat cover; I was now attending about three classes a week.

Finally, I thought, a gym activity where women can really be strong and fast and challenge the hegemonic fit female body that emerged in the late twentieth century. Finally, somewhere my thick muscled calves would be appreciated and challenged. Finally, a place where wearing spandex wasn't read as an invitation for ogling eyes. I looked forward to these classes, and I left them pleasantly soaked in sweat. Was this empowerment I was feeling? And is indoor cycling a potentially liberatory—more so than traditional aerobics—activity for women?

The inherent differences between indoor cycling and other forms of aerobics, some of which I mentioned earlier, also included the appeal to self-described uncoordinated people who worry about tripping over steps or being unable to master difficult, dancelike moves in a traditional aerobics class. There is also an element of individuality and privacy in the indoor cycling classroom. Though there are others in the room, only you know how high or low your resistance/tension dial is set. The competitive nature of the aerobics classroom and the surveillance facilitated by mirrored walls is mitigated in the indoor cycling room. The ability of the individual to privately control the intensity of the workout makes indoor cycling a better vehicle for empowerment. It is not, however, without its problems.

Right now it is perhaps physically empowering to some participants. I experienced this empowerment myself as a participant and have seen it as an instructor. But I have yet to witness or hear of an indoor cycling class that can engender the *mind-body* empowerment Castelnuovo and Guthrie write of that is, I believe, the ultimate goal of women's sport and physical activity. Many of the problems, though, can be mitigated through better instructor training, a commitment to creating a feminist environment, and an overall paradigm shift about group exercise. And these are the issues participants and instructors need to address before adequately assessing the empowerment potential of this activity.

When I left the East Coast and moved to the Midwest, I joined a gym I thought would be similar to my old one where I began cycling. But I entered a very different gym atmosphere. There were no literal walls, which often create gendered spaces, separating cardio equipment from weights (the former seen as feminine, the latter masculine).[3] But the gendered environment and expectations were palpable: slick advertisements for corporately created aerobics classes picturing thin, toned, glistening, tan women, a myriad of weight loss contests in which one could participate, and a homophobic atmosphere that manifests itself in varying degrees against queer members, some of whom have since left because they felt targeted by management. My ticker tape of discontent was streaming furiously, so I again sought refuge in the cycling room.

What follows are the observations I made as a participant-observer in one gym over the two years I took and taught indoor cycling.[4] Located in a mid-size college town in the Midwest, Fitness Barn[5] is a private gym that caters to middle- and upper-middle-class people, many of whom are affiliated with the University of Iowa. Members range in age from teenagers to senior citizens, and there is a fairly equal distribution of men and women. The majority of Fitness Barn members are white, reflecting state demographics. Within the indoor cycling classroom, it is more difficult to accurately describe the population due to the nature of the activity, which attracts a mix of regulars, infrequent cyclists, and the occasional one-timer. My initial observations suggest that the majority of cyclists are in their twenties, thirties, or forties. Most are women, but there are significantly more men in indoor cycling classes than in any other type of aerobics class offered at Fitness Barn—in the majority of classes there are always a handful of men.

These were the demographics I found when I entered my first class at my new gym several years ago now. This first experience was deeply disappointing. The instructor wore a floral cycling skort (skirt with attached padded cycling shorts). I tried to temper my initial reaction to what I perceived as an odd display of femininity in a very acceptable activity for women (in contrast to many recreational and institutional sports and even certain activities within the gym such as weight lifting during which women often must engage in overt displays of femininity). But I reminded myself that I too conform to certain gendered expectations when I don skirts to play tennis. So while I could accept skirt-wearing instructors, I was unable to stomach the (per)version of indoor cycling I experienced at my new gym. This first instructor was actually one of the least egregious, I discovered, only after trying almost every other instructor.

I have been in classes where the instructors have called us sissies, wusses, and wimps. One female instructor takes a very militaristic tone, accuses people of not working hard enough, not doing a drill correctly, using improper form, and, because of these things, wasting her time. She has been referred to as the Spin Nazi—jovially of course, but the problematic "title" indicates the level of intensity she creates in her class. In all fairness, her classes are almost always full. Her style is embraced by some members who say they want that type of motivation.[6] Most members who take indoor cycling classes are aware of the differing styles of instructors. Newcomers quickly, through experience and word of mouth, learn which instructors are most conducive to their own fitness goals. There are choices, and members can exert some degree of agency through them.

Styles differ among instructors, but pervasive among all of the instructors are the subtle comments, seemingly made with the best of intentions but in an uncritical manner, that reinforce a gendered and disempowering experience. Aerobics classes perpetuate a paradigm of group exercise that privileges weight loss over all other benefits of exercise. Despite the differences between aerobics and indoor cycling, the latter has not been immune to the emphasis on weight loss. Instructors engage in confessional moments, seemingly as a way to bond or break down the instructor-student barrier, while teaching, making comments such as "I ate a brownie last night, so I have to work hard this morning." Even instructors very conscious of letting participants control their own pace and level of intensity make comments such as "Let's work hard now so we can eat later." The use of the collective we is intended to be nonthreatening, an attempt not to single anyone out, yet it still presumes and perpetuates the belief that the primary motivation behind the workout is weight loss or maintenance.[7]

Heidi, whose classes are usually near or at capacity, is the instructor whose cycling pedagogy I admire and have drawn from the most. Her philosophy and style of cycling can meet the needs of variety of students, and this is evident in the members she attracts to her class. The age range is much wider in her classes than most: college students through senior citizens. Of note also is the range of fitness levels in her class. Whereas some of the more intense instructors attract only those who are already in above-average physical condition, the participants in Heidi's class fall along a wide spectrum of fitness levels, including beginning exercisers as well as competitive racers and triathletes.

Aspects of Heidi's teaching philosophy have the potential to empower all participants. At the start of each class and throughout she makes statements such as "This is your workout," or "Take it where you need to," and she offers modifications to alter the intensity in either direction. Rather than telling participants what they should be doing and at what level they should be doing it, she gives control of the workout back to her participants and serves more as an experienced guide. Heidi herself always works hard in class, and so she serves as an example, but without suggesting that everyone needs to be working as hard as she does. She does not disparage anyone who chooses not to work at that same level of intensity.

But even Heidi can negate the empowering possibilities of the activity. I was very surprised one day to hear her add to the instruction to take it to the next level *if you want*: "It depends on how much damage you want to do to yourself today." Whether she was aware of it or not (I suspect not), she reified the common yet harmful "no pain, no gain" philosophy that permeates almost all aspects of sport and training. Certainly it is ubiquitous at the higher levels of institutional sport (and it is increasingly present in high school and youth sport, perpetuated by overly competitive coaches and parents), and it has become an unexamined aspect of gym culture.

This statement, in the gendered space of the indoor cycling studio, can be read more insidiously as reinforcing the need, for women especially, to adopt masochistic tendencies in order to measure their levels of success. Bordo says: "Food refusal, weight loss, commitment to exercise, and ability to tolerate bodily pain and exhaustion have become cultural metaphors for self-determination, will and moral fortitude" (2003, 681). I don't want to do any damage[8] to myself today, I thought. And then I questioned, throughout that day what that meant about my commitment to exercise, to my own fitness, and to my ability as a woman to achieve "success"—however abstractly constructed and measured.

Other instructors perpetuate the weight loss paradigm of exercise, and the holidays are the worst time of year. In Heidi's class, two days before Thanksgiving, there was an unusual amount of weight loss/weight maintenance rhetoric. Twice she told us to "drink a tall glass of water and eat a small salad or bowl of soup" before the meal so we would be partially full when we sat down to eat and thus, presumably, avoid some kind of uncontrolled gorging to which we would otherwise fall prey. The goal of that class—one she repeated several times—was to work off what we hadn't yet eaten: the apple pie, the mashed potatoes with gravy, and other such dishes that she made a point to name.

This rhetoric is so pervasive that the illogical nature of a comment like the one Heidi made is barely perceptible—how can one work off what one has not yet consumed? This kind of atmosphere, which is not unusual to my gym, is the main impediment to empowerment or any other liberatory experience in indoor cycling. Certainly instructors as individuals have not created the cultural climate that explicitly links exercise to weight loss, but the fitness industry as a whole has "both benefited from and incited women's preoccupation with weight control" (Cahn 1994, 274). Instructors are implicated in this statement, and members who join gyms with the primary goal of losing weight are encouraged by instructors who talk excessively about shedding pounds, counting calories, and burning fat.

It is difficult, if not impossible, to alter the fitness industry's marketing strategies that promote gyms through implicit and explicit promises of drastic weight loss. And instructors must recognize that the majority of women who join are motivated by these promises. But this does not mean women have to instruct under the limits of this paradigm. Though I believe that weight loss can create some form of empowerment, it cannot occur unless the process itself offers some form of empowerment. Group exercise instructors are integral in creating an atmosphere in which all of their participants—regardless of their reason for being in the class[9]—can enjoy and succeed.

Instructors are pivotal in the process of creating an emotionally and a physically healthy environment that has the potential to empower. Markula argues in her study of aerobics participants that the experience is neither inherently empowering nor disempowering (2003, 55). Many of the informants in her ethnography of female aerobicizers attest that participants and instructors engage in resistant practices as a means of accessing empowerment (70–71). Markula, though, is concerned that the complexity of modern power relations makes it difficult even to discern what constitutes resistance and empowerment (74). I do not wish to simplify these concerns here and certainly agree with Markula that the complexity of power dynamics present in the gym requires further investigation. But I do not think this negates a consideration of how a commitment to a feminist pedagogy in indoor cycling can begin to constitute a strategy of resistance.

My construction and practice of a feminist pedagogy of indoor cycling involves both rather simple modifications as well as more radical practices that would necessarily involve a dramatic alteration in how group exercise is conceived and executed in the contemporary American gym. They all constitute a critical feminist pedagogy that I have tried to implement but that remains fluid to better accommodate the needs of my own students.

The genesis of my conception of a feminist pedagogy of indoor cycling actually came at an unusual entry point: the music. Unlike aerobics, where instructors use music engineered specifically for these classes, cycling instructors make their own mixes.[10] The right sound track can make or break a class. As a participant I have had to cycle through peppy, motivating music that has misogynist overtones. I am exasperated at being told over and over to "Whip it! Whip it good!" or "Push it—push it real hard" and by songs that sexualize women's "booties" and "racks." I labor over my playlists, agonizing over whether including songs such as the Dixie Chicks' "Cowboy Take Me Away" or a cover of "I Need a Hero" could be disempowering because of the women-in-need-of-rescue theme. I love the beat of Eminem's tracks but worry about the homophobia and misogyny. I took Ram Jam's "Black Betty" out of my usual rotation when I found out the NAACP has deemed it racist and misogynist. Music can set the tone of a class, and the feedback I receive indicates that the music selection heavily influences participants' preferences in instructors.

In short, instructors have a rapt audience that is listening closely to what comes over the speakers. Feminists have long known that language matters. It is just as important to pay attention when that language is set to music. The lyrics are important because they can correspond or contradict the messages instructors are sending. I try to be hyperaware of the ways I am trying to motivate during class. I never mention food consumption or fat and calorie burning. My encouragements to "work hard" are never followed by "so you don't have to feel guilty about last night's dessert." Rather than saying something like "This drill will make your thighs firm," I use phrasing that puts the emphasis on what participants should be feeling when they do it: "You should be using your quads and hamstrings here," or, "You'll feel this in your glutes." Like Heidi, I frequently suggest modifications to allow all levels of cyclists to participate at their ability level. These purposeful comments could easily be negated by a pop singer extolling the virtues of a tight derriere.

I have constructed my pedagogy in such a way as to provide participants a certain amount of agency. Also, part of my larger project is breaking down the hierarchy that exists between instructor and participant. I teach indoor cycling from a raised platform—literally on a higher level than participants.[11] While I see the practicality of this—allowing all to see what the instructor is doing—it creates a false power dynamic. I see myself as a guide, and I say this at the start of my classes. But sometimes this concept too becomes abstract. I would like to be able to establish a better feedback system where participants can (anonymously if they wish) suggest drills that I can incorporate into workouts. This gives them a greater stake in the class and begins to disrupt some of the notions that instructors are all-knowing and that participants are only receptacles.

These are practices in which I already engage or would not find difficult to implement. But more resistant practices are available to me that might begin to change the philosophy of indoor cycling to make it more conducive to an empowering and a liberatory practice.

The first few minutes of my class—and all others I have taken—consists of a warm-up to prevent muscle injury. But what about our minds? Yoga, as well as other mindful practices, explicitly eschews a Cartesian duality, but in indoor cycling we rarely consider our mental energy, even as we put our bodies through an intense physical experience. In an attempt to deconstruct this binary, Haravon Collins incorporated aspects of mindful practices in her aerobics classes. It would not be difficult to do the same in indoor cycling. A brief (three minutes or so) period where we are lightly cycling on our bikes with eyes closed and quiet or with no music can help instructors and participants assess their whole selves. If instructor training programs incorporated this kind of interdisciplinarity, then instructors could—as mindful practice instructors do—guide participants through a process of setting goals, noticing sore or tired parts of their body, and taking stock of what feels good.

Also during this time instructors can instill a sense of focus. For example, at the start of most yoga classes, instructors tell participants to "stay in the room" by thinking only about themselves (which also discourages competition) and their workout for the duration of the class.

This encourages participants to release stress related to their "outside" lives—part of the reason many people exercise in the first place.

Such practices have their genesis in the critical feminist consciousness that I have developed inside and outside of the gym. A feminist pedagogy in indoor cycling begins by engendering a critical consciousness in instructors. Instructors need to be aware of the messages they are sending with their comments—all intended to be encouraging, though not always received thusly—their music, and their practices and behaviors in class.

Markula warns that it is dangerous to assume that women's resistant practices and increased presence in fitness activities can adequately challenge the structures that have historically disempowered women (2003, 74). I share these hesitations, but as someone who is now part of the system through my position as an instructor, I cannot eschew the challenge presented to me to work toward a more empowering practice and, ultimately, a less patriarchal gym experience. Using instructors as a starting point for challenging fitness industry hegemony allows for the possibility of change in many directions.

Notes

1. The space of the gym and the members who enter it are of course raced and classed and marked in numerous other ways that all intersect and construct the gendered body. While I have a deep epistemological commitment to revealing these intersections as they exist in the gym and in sport, my experiences to date have been in gyms that are relatively homogenous in terms of race, class, and sexuality. But throughout this chapter, where possible, I have included stories and analyses pertaining to the raced, able-bodied, and heternormalized atmosphere in the gym.

2. Often the term *spin* is used as a shorthand for indoor cycling (i.e., I am going to spin class, or I am going spinning), but "Spin" is actually a trademark of Reebok and refers to its specific indoor cycling program. I use indoor cycling and cyclists throughout this chapter because I am referring to the activity in general, not a specific corporate program.

3. Johnston (1998) offers an excellent analysis of how the literal spaces within a gym are marked by gendered boundaries that limit a woman's access to activities such as weight lifting that have the potential to desexualize and empower.

4. Since the end of this period I have moved back to the East Coast and continue to teach indoor cycling in a gym with similar demographics but a slightly different atmosphere due, I suspect, to the more liberal town and region in which I live. Observations that I have made in this new space

that run counter or significantly contribute to my initial ones are included as endnotes.

5. The name of this business and the names of all members and instructors have been changed.

6. I am intrigued by such unquestioned styles of motivation, which are drawn from coaching methods and border on abuse at times. They are not my focus here, but further inquiry into how and when these motivational techniques—accepted in men's sports and now in many levels of competitive women's sports—have entered the gym is necessary as we continue to explore the dominant ideologies perpetuated in the gym.

7. The perpetuation of the weight-loss rhetoric in indoor cycling classes illustrates just how ingrained it has become. A quick look at the participants shows that many are competitive athletes (marathoners, runners, triathletes, and so on) using the class for training purposes. They would never claim to be using the class for weight-loss purposes.

8. I realize that physiological "damage" occurs whenever I exercise, in the form of muscle breakdown that leads to rebuilding. This process is not the one Heidi was referencing in her statement. Hers was suggestive of a more intense physical experience that would result in painful after effects.

9. Markula (2003) and Haravon Collins (2002), in their ethnographies of female aerobic students, found that many do not necessarily enter the activity for the sole purpose of losing weight, though they are always negotiating the contradictory messages regarding fitness, weight loss, appropriate femininity, and sexuality that women receive in the gym.

10. Some indoor cycling programs have been developed by corporations that include ready-made drills and music, but they are far from the norm in indoor cycling.

11. In my current situation, there is no platform. I have found that allows for greater dialogue—both playful and serious (asking questions about form or technique)—between myself and those in my class.

Works Cited

Bordo, Susan. 2003. *Unbearable Weight: Feminism, Western Culture, and the Body.* Berkeley: University of California Press.

Bourdieu, Pierre. 1984. *Distinction: A Social Critique of the Judgement of Taste.* London: Routledge.

Cahn, Susan. 1994. *Coming on Strong: Gender and Sexuality in Twentieth-Century Women's Sport.* Cambridge, MA: Harvard University Press.

Castelnuovo, Shirley, and Sharon R. Guthrie. 1998. *Feminism and the Female Body: Liberating the Amazon Within.* Boulder, CO: Lynne Rienner.

Haravon Collins, Lesley. 1995. "Exercises in Empowerment: Toward a Feminist Aerobic Pedagogy." *Women in Sport and Physical Activity Journal* 4: 23–44.

the muscular woman out of the context of the gym. In doing so, they remove her from an important group setting where she engages in a process that has the potential to build body, mind, and community.

The History of Muscular Female Types:
The Superhuman Strongwoman
and the Well-Built Bombshell

From a historical perspective, we see that these two types—the sporting woman of advertising culture and the hypermuscular woman of bodybuilding—constitute a pair that can be tracked through the history of weight training, from the early margins of the sideshow to the contemporary mainstream gym. In America, women's bodybuilding began in the late nineteenth century under the big top, where strongwomen were expected to challenge the prevailing standards (as does the more recent hypermuscular bodybuilder). But since the turn of the last century, bodybuilding has also been marketed to middle-class women as a standardizing procedure—an activity enabling them to better fit the prevailing standards of beauty (as does our current fitness icon). So, from a historical perspective, the hypermuscular type derives from the earliest sideshow strongwomen, who carried men on their shoulders, dangled weights from their teeth, and caught cannonballs with their bare hands. Meanwhile, the more traditionally attractive type follows in the footsteps of the hoards of women at the beginning of the twentieth century who began weight training to perfect their figures at the advice of bodybuilder entrepreneurs Eugen Sandow and Bernarr MacFadden. Sandow and MacFadden marketed bodybuilding to a broad clientele—including men, women, and children of the middle and upper classes. As a result, the reputation of bodybuilding shifted from a peculiar practice for sideshow characters and seedy activity for working-class men to a respectable "science" and popular trend of "physical culture" for the growing middle class. Indeed, the familiar sporting woman icon currently gracing the glossy pages of so many major magazines is a sign that the female muscularity endorsed by Sandow and MacFadden over 100 years ago has been successfully normalized by the now-large and lucrative industries of health, fitness, and beauty.

Since Sandow and McFadden, however, the identity of bodybuilding as an industry and a practice has remained stuck between the margins of the sideshow and the mainstream marketplace. Today's female (and male) bodybuilders, albeit often unknowingly, remain caught at a

cross road: one turn takes them back toward the subversive stages of
vaudeville, where they once were expected to surpass human limitations, while the other turn moves them in the direction of mainstream
ideals, where they serve as the models of human perfection. This split
personality of bodybuilding explains the visible contradictions embodied
by today's professional female bodybuilders. Their hypermuscularity
holds true to their historical roots as groundbreaking strongwomen,
while their hyperfeminine accoutrement works to fashion them as
exemplars of beauty. It also helps explain the bifurcation of muscular
types that we see in our media today. We can already locate this bifurcation of types on the stages of vaudeville in the famous characters of
Minerva (circa 1890s) and Sandwina (circa 1920s).

Two Strongwomen of Vaudeville

At 5'8" and over 220 pounds, Josie Wohlford cut an intimidating figure
as Minerva, America's first famous strongwoman. In the 1890s, several
years before Sandow began selling bodybuilding as a popular activity
of health and beauty, Minerva received widespread publicity for her
astounding feats of strength. Her most famous accomplishment was
a "hip and harness lift" done at the Bijou Theatre in Hoboken, New
Jersey. During her act, the hulking strongwoman allegedly lifted eighteen men on a platform for a total lift of over 3,000 pounds, setting
the Guinness Book of World Records for the greatest weight lifted by
a woman and receiving a specially made championship belt from the
Police Gazette—the most important sporting tabloid of the time.[1]
    While Minerva was recognized for her massive build, awesome
strength, and temperamental personality, it was not simply these
"mannish" qualities that constituted her subversive stature. In an 1893
lithograph, Minerva appears in the posture and attire of a strongman.
She wears an androgynous, leopard skin, gladiator-like outfit, and her
hair is either short or fastened so closely to her neck that it gives the
appearance of being short. With one arm, the strongwoman holds
a barbell on its side while stomping, with one foot, on the ball of
another barbell. The assertion of power represented by Minerva's "I
came, I saw, I conquered" stance recalls the classical statues of heroic
athletes. Such imaging, replete with its foregrounded view of Minerva's
bicep, is quite similar to the stock images of popular strongmen that
circulated at approximately the same time.
    Twenty years after the "physical culture" craze, which was
spawned by Sandow and cultivated by MacFadden, had swept America,

a different type of strongwoman appeared. The "New Woman" of vaudeville was Katie Brumbach Heyden, who took Sandwina as her stage name. Borrowing not only Sandow's name but also his reputation as a model of human splendor, Sandwina became the main attraction for the Ringling Brothers Circus in 1910. Unlike the awesome Minerva, with her blocky frame, Sandwina was admired (and probably also desired) for her hourglass figure, comely face, and elegant mannerisms. She was billed as the "Beautiful Herculean Venus," not only the "strongest woman that ever lived" but also the one "possessing the most perfect feminine" form. In the colorful circus posters advertising Sandwina's act, gone are the stock strongman poses and strongman outfits seen in the depictions of Minerva. Instead, Sandwina appears in bucolic surroundings and resembles a cross between a pinup star and a ballerina. Wearing a revealing body suit, ballet tights, and high-heeled boots, Sandwina flirtatiously cocks one hand under her chin and delicately points her toes. Red roses and pink ribbons frame her statuesque form. Overall, the representations of Minerva emphasized her superhuman strength, while those of Sandwina revealed her beguiling beauty: the muscular babe was born.

Media Babes Pudgy Stockton and Babe Didrikson

While Sandwina marks the emergence of a sexy strongwoman type in America, the mainstream spread of the muscular babe really begins in the late 1930s with the rise of Abbye "Pudgy" Stockton—America's golden girl beach performer. With her silver- blonde hair, wholesome good looks, and sizeable bust, Stockton embodies a shift in the imaging of muscle-built women, partly due to the wider circulation of physique magazines (such as Bob Hoffman's *Strength and Health*) and the wider availability of weight-training equipment (such as Hoffman's York Barbells). Stockton became famous for her exceptional physique, with its 38-20-36 measurements (Rose 2001, 46) as well as her spectacular beachside acrobatic and tumbling performances. She drew so many spectators to Santa Monica Beach that the town eventually erected a public stage there, inaugurating the original Muscle Beach. With Stockton, the girl-next-door acrobat of the public beach supplanted the daunting strongwoman of the vaudeville sideshow. In contrast to earlier strongwomen, America's new type of muscular woman combined strength, health, and *glamour*. Stockton underscored her favorable status as a babe with biceps through constant association with her acrobatic partner-husband. She also insisted on the cosmetic benefits of barbell training and the fashion-ableness of muscles.

One common type of publicity photo shows Stockton at Muscle Beach poised as the striking centerpiece of a four-person strength act. She sports a rosy complexion and the mid-length hairdo of Hollywood stars. On her petite (5'1") but voluptuous frame, Stockton wears a flowered, two-piece bathing suit, considered risqué by the conservative standards of her day. In the pivotal position of the "under stander," Stockton holds her husband up over her head. She smiles prettily and stands resolutely, supporting him as he rises like a rocket into cloud-less blue skies. In spite of Stockton's apparent strength, such images of her buttress the conventional wisdom of the era. Read metaphori-cally, photographs such as these suggest that men soar effortlessly on the backs of solid self-sacrificing women. In fact, Stockton stopped flexing her biceps for photographers because she did not want to be seen as competing with men. More superficially, these images show that women can be both muscular and sexy.

For her conventional looks and traditional choices, Stockton was abundantly rewarded. She received widespread media attention, appearing on the cover of forty-two magazines and in hundreds of other publications, including *Life, Pic*, and *Laff*. If Sandwina was the first muscular babe to personally capitalize on her sexy appearance, then Stockton was the first muscular bombshell to sell to other women the feminine sex appeal of muscles. As part of her campaign to promote female muscularity, Stockton coined the term "athletic femininity" in her magazine column "Barbelles," which appeared in *Strength and Health*. She also sold the cosmetic benefits of weight training in her own Los Angeles-based all-women's gym. At her "Salon of Figure Develop-ment," which specialized in "Bust Development, Figure Contouring, and Reducing," Stockton helped women weight train in order to look good in clothes—to "have a small waist and a flat tummy" (Frueh 1999, 153). A long line of petite, conventionally attractive bodybuilders—from Lisa Lyon (who actually trained with Stockton), to Rachel McLish, to any of today's Miss Olympia Fitness or Figure competitors—emulates Stockton in building sexy, muscular bodies.

Of course, no discussion of important muscular babes of the 1930s and 1940s is complete without mentioning America's most famous babe of that time—Mildred "Babe" Didrikson. Didrikson was exhaustively publicized by the sports journalists of her era. The "Babe" became a household word, partly because of her freakish capacity to excel as a woman at so many sports, from running to boxing to golfing. (Babe actually did appear briefly on the stages of vaudeville as a freakish woman who could run fast on a treadmill.) Between the period 1930–1932, Didrikson held American, Olympic, or World records in five separate track and field events. A decade later, she continued her triumphant streak, winning eighty-two golf tournaments. But beyond her wide-ranging athletic accomplishments, Didrikson's legend involves a widely reported transformation of self and body type—from the subversive figure of an aggressive tomboy track-and-field athlete into a glamorous golfing lady.

As a young track and field star, Didrikson upset the status quo not only with her amazing athleticism but also with her gender-bending appearance. News articles of the era commonly fixated on her unconventional looks—her short hair, strong jaw, wiry muscles, and boyish attire. Journalists also noted her unconventional personality—her declared indifference toward men, reputed wrath toward fellow competitors, and confessed capacity to eat large amounts of food.[2]

Only five years later, Didrikson transformed into a sophisticated businesswoman golfer. She accomplished this change of image partly with the help of swank clothing and fashionable accessories: her "pretty hats" made headlines. Didrikson also married a famous wrestler and, like Stockton, routinely appeared publicly with him. *Life* magazine cheerfully announced her self-transformation in the headline: "Babe Is a Lady Now: The World's Most Amazing Athlete Has Learned How to Cook and Care for Her Huge Husband" ("Babe" 1947, 90). Babe's transformation, however, was also coded in her body through a frequently remarked upon change from a lean, flat-chested, muscular build to a new curvaceous figure with wider hips, larger breasts, and a smaller waistline.

While the remaking of Didrikson's image may have been partly the result of an organic process of physical maturation, it is clear that her womanly self-stylization achieved through marriage and fashion choices contributed to her success as a golfing star, particularly as it made her more acceptable to the country-club set running the sport. In this manner, she forecasts a similar tendency among today's hypermuscular female bodybuilders. Like Didrikson, female bodybuilders must work to contour their bodies and images so that they comply with the standards of a male-run industry. For instance, the International Federation of Bodybuilders (IFBB), which presides over the Ms. Olympia Bodybuilding Competition, still has rules regarding complexion, makeup, and jewelry. According to the IFBB, these rules ensure that their competitors will "conform to standards of taste and decency" (24). Bodybuilders who internalize the industry pressure and mind-set mitigate their extreme muscularity by feminizing their appearances. Also, like Didrikson, they often reject feminism and resist the opportunity to form a community with other female athletes.

The Face-off of *Pumping Iron II* Stars Rachel McLish and Bev Francis

The division of muscular types that I have been tracking was explicitly documented, forty years after Stockton and Babe, in George Butler's 1985 docudrama *Pumping Iron II: The Women.* In *Pumping Iron II,* Butler contrived and scripted a face-off between girly-girl bodybuilder Rachel McLish, the slender and leggy industry darling—and Bev Francis, a gender-bending Australian power lifter with levels of muscularity never before seen in a woman's bodybuilding event. Butler has claimed that he initially was uncertain if Francis was really a woman; nevertheless, he went to great lengths to get her to star in his film. He traveled to Australia to find her and then worked to convince her to come to America and train as a bodybuilder. Although the narrative of *Pumping Iron II* makes it seem as if Francis posed a serious threat to McLish, from an industry standpoint, it was quite clear that Francis would not win the bodybuilding competition featured in Butler's film. After all, she was a bulky powerlifter, not a chiseled bodybuilder, so her enormous proportions were far too controversial to appeal to the stodgy IFBB judges presiding over the event. Ultimately, Francis placed eighth but still emerged as an audience favorite. *Pumping Iron II* changed Francis's life permanently, launching her career as a professional bodybuilder. It also changed the face of professional bodybuilding permanently. From this point onward, vein-ridged, steroid-enhanced bodies began to dominate the stages of female bodybuilding contests.

In seeking out Bev Francis, Butler must have intuitively or overtly known that the two different muscular types going back to the hulking Minerva and comely Sandwina already existed in the cultural imagination, and that audiences would expect any movie on women's bodybuilding to feature both types. Certainly, the IFBB also must have been aware of this audience expectation when they created their new Miss Olympia Fitness and Miss Olympia Figure competitions to offset the steroid-built bodies that now overshadow professional bodybuilding events. Judges presiding over these newer competitions look for a combination of beauty and "aesthetic physique" and penalize athletes who display excessive muscularity.

After so many years of coexistence, the hypermuscular and sexy muscular types now depend upon each other for their survival. By virtue of their excessive muscularity, freaky strongwomen and hyper-muscular bodybuilders, such as Francis, carve out space for women with smaller muscles to appear "normal" (read: fashionable). Had the hypermuscular type that reaches back to Minerva not already charted the territory of female muscularity, the fit woman in the Nike ad would still seem unusual today. But the hypermuscular type epitomized by Francis also requires her stylish smaller sister for self-definition. Against this more normative type, the hypermuscular type can appear larger than life—a futuristic figure of female potency.

Our Bodies, Our Social Systems, Our Selves

What this history of the hypermuscular and sexy muscular types shows us is that today's proliferation of muscular female images is intrinsically linked to the commercial development of bodybuilding and its crossover into the profitable industries of health, beauty, and the body. For over 100 years, muscles, bodies, and "the self" have been seamlessly united in marketing strategies targeting women. Until now, "third-wave" feminist discussions of women in the gym have largely ignored this history. Armed with the New Age notion that "changing the self changes the world," these feminists focus on the freedom of self-expression. They claim that weight training and working out are revolutionary because they transform individual bodies, chang-ing the world one muscular woman at a time. This claim overlooks the fact that since the turn of the last century, weight training has been sold to women as a normalizing practice to achieve a standard look. Third-wave feminist arguments also construe the consumerist behaviors of gym culture as "free choices" and celebrate the stan-dardizing procedure of bodybuilding as transformational. Generally, these discussions overlook the conformist aspects of everyday gym life—from the dieting and agonizing over body fat, to the incessant scanning of other women's bodies, to the cooing over and competing for the hottest male personal trainer on the floor. They also ignore the disciplining aspects of the bodybuilder's regime: the food scales and eating schedules; diuretics, supplements, and steroids; and let's not forget the hours and hours of doing cardio and pumping iron.

Unfortunately, these celebrations of muscular women also fre-quently take them out of the context of the gym. In doing so, they remove them from an important communal practice. Gyms bring a variety of women together in small groups for activities that change individual bodies, but the collective work that occurs there has resulted in broader and more valuable changes in women's styles of representation and in social definitions of femininity. Hypermuscular female bodybuilders force us to question what it means to be a "natural woman." And all women who work out counter social constructs that conflate the concept of the feminine with that of the passive body. But in order to change more than our cultural metaphors, the questioning of gender norms that begins in the gym with the construction of strength and muscles must move out into the world to address systemic problems. Certainly, that so many gyms now sponsor events to raise money and awareness for important social causes—from the local money collections for the victims of Hurricane Katrina to the nation-wide Work Out for Hope project that benefits HIV/AIDS and related cancers research—is a hopeful sign that gym-going women can move beyond the goal of personal transformation to face the bigger challenge of changing social policy.

Carla Dunlap faces this challenge head on in *Pumping Iron II*. Dunlap, as I have argued elsewhere,[3] is important in the history of bodybuilding not only because she is the actual contest winner in Butler's movie but also because she is its feminist voice and communal force. In one poignant scene, Dunlap, flanked by her fellow female bodybuilders, confidently questions the IFBB judges on their definition of femininity. Here Dunlap demonstrates that the collective body forged by female bodybuilders has the potential to initiate the urgent discussions and ask the hard questions that can lead to policy changes. Juxtaposed against the peacockish Rachel McLish, who in the preceding scene snorts at the IFBB judges when they reject her padded bathing suit, Dunlap is a refreshing reminder that female bodybuilders are not only defined by their awesome appearances. By questioning the IFBB judges in this manner, Dunlap shows us that we are not simply "our muscular bodies/our powerful selves" but actually "our bodies, our social systems, our selves." This point is deeply resonant today as the *Roe v. Wade* decision grows ever more vulnerable in spite of the increasing number of women with powerful bodies.

Of course, having the free choice to forge a powerful body is not a bad thing. Nor for that matter is having access to an array of available merchandise that might support that choice. In general, however, I question the recent resurrection of the invincible body, even in the form of the muscular female. This valorization of the woman warrior troubles me because it recuperates the predominant concept of aggressive masculinity, enabling feminists to venerate misogynist bodybuilders such as Arnold Swarzenegger. By far the worst consequence of such unreflective celebrations of female stealth, however, can be seen in the photographs of Abu Graib prison, where American women torturers flexed their muscles for the camera to show their dominance over their helpless Iraqi victims.

But there is a hopeful new vision of muscular women today that goes beyond the lone images of the freakish strongwoman and well-built bombshell. Go to—better yet participate in—a walk for breast cancer. Look around at the crowd of sweaty walkers and the many smiling women who move together arm in arm. See how they lean into and support each other. At first pass, several of these women could belong in an ad for a beauty product or sportswear line, except that some of them wear a baseball cap with the word "survivor" stitched in bright white letters across the front. With this bold marking, these women indirectly caution us that in an unstable world neither our individuated bodies nor our individual selves are dependable sources of power. More reliable strength lies in the vigorous gathering of women whose collective energy is mobilized in a work out and *the work for* social change.

Notes

1. This section on Minerva draws on the work of bodybuilding historian Jan Todd. See Todd 1990.

2. Newspapers also noted Minerva's unusual capacity to consume large quantities of food.

3. Although Dunlap has been construed as the safe middle ground between McLish and Francis, I argue that she is actually the most radical choice for a contest winner because she stands in as a communal force and connects to a history of African-American activism. See Brady 2000.

Works Cited

"Babe Is a Lady Now: The World's Most Amazing Athlete Has Learned How to Cook and Care for Her Huge Husband." 1947. *Life* 23 (June): 90.

Brady, Jacqueline. 2000. "Pumping Iron with Resistance: Carla Dunlap's Victorious Body." In *Recovering the Body: Self-representations by African American Women*, ed. Michael Bennett and Vanessa Dikerson, 253–78. New Brunswick, NJ: Rutgers University Press.

Butler, George. 1985. *Pumping Iron II: The Women*. Film. Directed by George Butler. Distributed by Blue Dolphin Film and Cinecom International Films.

Frueh, Joanna. 1999. "Interview with Pudgy Stockton." In *Picturing the Modern Amazon*, ed. Joanna Frueh, Laurie Fierstein, and Judith Stein, 152–54. New York: Rizzoli.

IFBB Rulebook. 2006. (October 29). International Federation of Bodybuilding and Fitness. April 12, 2009. http://www.ifbb.com/amarules/IFBBRulebook_2006-2007Edition.pdf.

Rose, Marl Matzer. 2001. *Muscle Beach: Where the Best Bodies in the World Started a Fitness Revolution.* New York: St. Martin's Griffin.

Todd, Jan. 1990. "The Mystery of Minerva." *Iron Game History* 1:2: 14–17.

7

Enduring Images

Catherine Houser

The woman on the elliptical machine has purple hands. Jamella comes to the gym every morning to try to get her joints moving, to try to stay a step ahead of her rheumatoid arthritis. She never complains about it, rarely ever talks about it. When I ask how she's managing now that they've taken her arthritis drug off the market, she holds up her left hand, swollen, painfully purple, and barely able to hold on to the handle on the elliptical machine, and she says it just means she'll have to work out a little longer each day to loosen up while she deals with the pain. They talk about the triathlete's ability to endure, but this, this is endurance.

I live in a small town on Cape Cod and I work out nearly every morning in a gym owned by a woman, though it is certainly not a "ladies gym." Most of the men and women there working out in the predawn hours are, like Jamella, old enough to be my parents. We see each other at the gym around the same time every morning. I'm part of a collection of women who come and go in their own way and on their own time, though very often in the same pattern of activity. We smile, we nod, we step out of the way when one or the other is passing in the narrow corridor on the way to the cardio deck. Then, once there, we plug in our headphones and focus on one of the twelve televisions lining the wall in front of us.

In that early morning dance, we have these little five-minute conversations where we learn of families, jobs, dogs, boats, political leanings, sports loyalties, vacations, and gardens, and when we're at a loss for words, we talk about the weather. It is an odd intimacy, knowing so much about these women's lives yet at the same time not even knowing their last names. But that is the nature of our relationship. We know each other in the gym where, very often, women of a certain age are working out other things besides their muscles, working toward something more than just a healthy body. What I found there in these half-sleepy, half-grumpy women was a road map for the rest of my life.

I lost my lifelong model for perseverance and endurance when my mother died shortly after I turned forty. I didn't know it at that moment, but when I lost my mother, I lost my way. Though my mother was no role model for physical health—she had five kids, an alcoholic husband, worked nights, and smoked two packs a day—she was my model for endurance. When she was suddenly gone and I was facing this broad morass of middle age, I found myself looking for someone to lead the way.

I didn't consciously go looking for someone. In fact, being one of those middle-age, half-grumpy women in the gym in the early morning, I am often annoyed by people I encounter. I am there to stave off the ravages of age, to manage an often out-of-control perimenopause, and to work out, quietly in my head, all of the prickly relationships that come with being the chair of an English Department. That's quite an agenda to tackle at 6 a.m. every morning. But I began to notice how much better I felt walking out of the gym on the days when I saw Jamella, Amy, Rosemary, and the others and we had one of our five-minute encounters.

As women, we often come to understand ourselves in the context of others. They become part of the story we tell ourselves. As young women, we measure ourselves, our bodies, against the women on the treadmill next to us. There is a competitiveness even in the simplest forms of fitness and health. Later, after we've played out our biological imperative, the women on the treadmill next to us are less our competition and more our comrades. So when I see Jamella, her eyes swollen, day after day for more than a week, I ask her if she's okay. She tells me her sister is dying of liver cancer. We exchange a few words, her trying to contain her sadness, me trying to find an expression of sympathy for this woman who I know but don't know. Then we each get on our elliptical machine, plug our earphones in, and stare at the row of televisions in front of us. I can feel the heaviness, the sadness, as she seems to just be going through the motions. And I feel myself working harder, faster than normal as if pulling her along, even though we're in our own space with our own thoughts. I think of my own little sister, now in her late forties, and I work even harder. On this day, I am soaked with sweat, as Jamella, having put in her time, is stepping down from the machine and collecting her things. "It won't always be this hard," I say to her. She smiles a half smile and says, "I hope you're right." She rarely misses a day during that ordeal. And the days turn into a year, and though it takes a while, I watch as the heaviness lifts, and she begins to work on the machines with intent, and her smile grows more real. I tell myself, remember this, this is how to survive great loss.

Over the years, some version of that story has happened again and again, yet through the trials we all keep rolling in in the predawn hours, finding the safety of a community of women without having the burden of commitment. When Alma, an eighty-two-year-old woman with a shock of white hair and purple T-shirt and tights, disappears for a couple of weeks, we ask each other if anyone has seen her. No one knows her last name, so we have no idea how to check up on her. We wait. When she appears a month later, she tells us her husband had a heart attack and she had to stay home tending to him, but now that he's able to be alone, she says, she "just had to get out." So she came back to the gym. She looks tight and slow as she starts out on the stationary bike, and when I say something about how tough it is getting back to working out, she says, "You have no idea—wait till you're my age." Her blue eyes twinkle. "The trick is, never quit." After she does her twenty minutes of cardio, she goes to lift weights—five-pound hand weights—and I watch her counting the reps, fully engaged, like it was her first time.

When I tell the story of my life to my friends, the women at the gym rarely ever appear in the narrative. Yet on days when I don't have to go to work, they are very often the only people I see or talk to. They don't know it, but I am constantly learning from them. I look for what I might look like at the gym at age sixty or seventy. Women of a certain age often become invisible to people. I watch them negotiate the space between the musclemen and the old men, and I notice how they claim their space. I see them roll their eyes with dismay at the tattooed young women, then catch them in awe when they see what these young and powerful women can do. I can see myself there, twenty years from now, and, as it is for most women going to the gym at any age, you have to be able to see yourself there before you can be comfortable there. I pay attention because I want to remember that this is possible.

8

The Gymnastics Group

Marcia Woodard

I.

Women are divided into two groups at an early age: tumblers and nontumblers.

In middle school, thick blue mats stretched out in parallel lines across the gym. Girls, aligned in twin columns, in spacious, hospital-blue, snap-up-the-front gym suits, waited their turn behind the blue lines. The skinny girls rolled up the legs and arms of their suits to sex them up.

I squatted and faced my classmates, my gym suit unaltered, and positioned myself for a series of backward somersaults. Momentum building: I rocked on the balls of my feet, pushed my fingertips into the mat, took deep preparatory breaths. The last thing I saw before letting go were the girls' watching faces. My left arm crumpled at the critical midway point. My head, not getting the clearance it needed, followed to the left at a potentially paralyzing angle. My legs and the rest of me also deviated left—as if somebody had let the air out of that side of my body—and I ended up on my hands and knees on the hardwood floor. Thump of a flat tire. The flush of embarrassment. My position completely dashed any hopes for consecutive somersaults.

I'm still not sure why I failed. I wonder if I feared performing the somersaults correctly because things would move too fast, because of my discomfort with dizzy.

I checked to see if anyone watched me after I fell off the mat. No. Their focus shifted. I hoped a few classmates would be "laughing with me, not at me" and I could ham it up for them. If the teacher looked busy, I duck-walked backwards down the mat—as if perpetually ready to start another somersault—and jumped up and ended my nonroutine with a hands-over-the-head, self-consoling Olympic flourish.

My body did not have a good working relationship with the cartwheel either. I tried out for cheerleader in middle school, and I'm sure I lost on the cartwheels. You know a good cartwheel: slow-motion spokes of a wheel. Hand, hand, leg, leg. My cartwheel, however, achieved successful symmetry only in the opening stance: both hands over my head like a "Y," legs spread, and rocking motion to accumulate compressed energy—or, rather, potential energy soon to go awry. I held the position for a long time, working up courage and positive visualization, pointing my face toward the desired trajectory, smelling my own sweat. Unfortunately, when my first hand contacted the floor, the momentum transferred to my posterior. My rear end assumed cartoonlike control and whipped my legs around at an angle that suggested broken knees. I ended up on the ground and tasted sour adrenaline in my throat. At the eighth-grade cheerleading tryouts, when I looked up to check the judges, they checked their notes. Later, I realized I should have known. Have you ever noticed how many movie stars are former cheerleaders? People watch them.

Headstands. I had to execute them against a wall. Without a wall, I got as far as resting my knees on my quivering elbows. My family called this knees-on-elbows maneuver "The Elephant Stand" because elephants performed this trick in the circus. I pulled out the half-stand only in the privacy of my backyard, and it guaranteed a good laugh; I could count on my family. Now, as an adult with friends who practice yoga, I've discovered my maneuver was a bastardized version of the "tripod" position. Of course. The original is something graceful to watch.

I eventually found a move I mastered. Not tumbling per se, more like a back-stretching exercise, but close enough. You lie on your back, put your palms on the floor next to your head, and push up with your arms and legs: you make an upside-down "U" with your body. I could "U." When I was around friends, I announced my back needed adjustment and lay on the floor and performed the "U" as part of the conversation circle. They had to look at me. And when they watched, I got a sense of being a tumbler. I was inside out, upside down, and so was the world. My hair hung down, fluid, swept the floor. My heart pulsed in my head. For a moment, I felt a part of the other group.

II.

I like to feel grounded. The back arch requires four limbs on the ground, but I still get the head rush. Grounded and ungrounded. Like electricity. Grounded has three pins, while ungrounded has two—makes sense. Four of my pins on the ground are best. What happens when I'm ungrounded? Is it like a shock? Haywire. With grounded it's safe, steady. The definition of grounded: "Intentionally connected to earth through a ground connection or connections . . . to prevent the buildup of voltages that may result in undue hazards to equipment or to persons" (http://www.wikipedia.com). The ground or earth is the conductor that exists primarily to help protect against faults. We're talking self-preservation. No blind faith. No leap of faith. Weightlessness, no. Grounded, yes.

III.

I avoided gymnastic-like voltages that might cause undue hazard to my person and participated in sports that didn't have watching or the defiance of gravity as a key component. I went interior. That's not to say I became a complete geek. I'm not making an appeal for sympathy (okay, maybe a little), but I realized that I would never place a checkmark next to cheerleader or student council (lost that race in eighth grade: "Come out of your tree and vote Marcia for VP"), and that I should redirect my talents.

High school. My sophomore year commenced in the fall of 1971; Title IX wouldn't pass until the following June. My chemistry partner, Laurel, a senior about half my size who brought brownies on lab days, encouraged me to turn out for the newly formed girl's cross-country team. The requirement of doggedness and running long distances through the woods where people couldn't see you attracted me. I found myself appreciated by and appreciating the long haul. Slow and steady running endorphins provided a head rush.

In cross-country meets, the starting line is also the finish line. A few people cheered us on at the start and did the same when we circled back around. I have no idea what spectators did while we were out on the course, and they had no idea what I did. The cheerleaders never came to our meets because they were watching football. Being a runner was the first time (maybe not exactly) I embraced an "otherness" and a disdain for the mainstream.

Our lack of status boosted team camaraderie, which revolved around eating. We ran and then we ate, or vice versa. If running is x and food is y, then x equals y. I loved the team pizza parties at Pizza Hut and picking black olives off slices and getting our money's worth from "all you can eat." One Saturday morning, before driving over the mountains to the state meet, we sat at two picnic tables in the coach's basement and ate pancakes cooked on a green Coleman camping stove. My mom made chocolate Halloween cupcakes with orange frosting and mellowcreme pumpkins on top for the division championships, and I passed them out on the bus after we lost the meet. Sometimes on training days, we rode to the local park squeezed into the PE teacher's station wagon, and stopped for Dairy Queen ice cream cones on the way back to school. I usually sat in the third seat that looked out the back window, licked the swirls smooth, and observed covered ground.

We ran in the rustle of autumn leaves along paths that bordered Seattle's Woodland Park Zoo. We ran out in the weather. Sweat equity stained my bra and stung my eyes: releasing versus keeping it in. Running hills next to the cemetery and timing our progress between tombstones. The smell of asphalt, dirt, grass, and exhaust on busy streets. My limbs brushed wet tree limbs. Rocks knocked in my pockets for barking dogs. Our shoe choices were two: white leather Nikes with the red swoosh (designed and debuted in 1971), or white leather Adidas with three green stripes. We ran at night with no fear and headlights in our eyes. We crawled on our knees and looked for Dana's contact lens in the grass. We gathered around gray gym lockers: click of the handle, spin of the Master lock. Blue sweats with white zippers. We stretched together in a circle on the grass. Shin splints: definitely grounded.

Between the beginning of track season my junior year and the end of cross-country season my senior year, I ran 1,000 miles. My blue and gold sweatshirt with the winged Shoreline Spartan and 1,000 Mile Club logo lives in my top dresser drawer. I worked as a dishwasher in an Alaskan fish camp that summer and ran six a day on the only homemade dirt road in Chignik Lagoon that connected the camp to the airstrip. If I ran down the gravel airstrip to the waves at the far end, and then up the grass trail to the wooden water reservoir on the creek behind camp, I covered 1.5 miles each direction. I ran while the wind blew the rain horizontally, my yellow fisherman's southwester tied under my chin. The fresh air smelled like snow. I ran in fear of bear but only encountered Missy, the camp St. Bernard. I flushed out ptarmigan that scared me with their sudden flapping: they blended with the summer-browned tundra. I relieved myself on the side of the road, and my waste was mistaken for bear droppings by the accountant's wife who went for an afternoon walk. I was voted most inspirational that fall. Covering new ground.

IV.

I've attempted yoga several times in the past ten years because my posture benefits and because the inward focus makes me less anxious about being watched. The problem is the ground is very far away. Yoga is "touch your palms to the floor" when my fingertips strain to reach mid-calf; it's recognizing that when I hold my foot one inch off the ground, my lack of balance may land me on my ass; and it's blood pooling in places my eighty-three-year-old mother believes are unhealthy: "You could hurt yourself." Yoga is déjà vu to gymnastics and a disabling lack of flexibility. I always need straps and several Styrofoam bricks for support, and I can't sit in that supposed relaxed, beginning position—the mislabeled Sit Easy position—without getting a backache. My breath gets shallow from the pain, and my lower back has a tantrum of cramps. I eventually give up and curl over like the top of a wave. Others may not watch me, but I watch them. I hate the sight of other women who *do* sit easy: erect, zoned out, and making that circle with their thumbs and forefingers while their hands rest on their knees. The circle is called a Mudra. The women make a Mudra because magnetic and electrical forces emanate from the tips of the fingers, and when the fingers are joined, an electrical circle is formed inside the body. Electricity that's circling and not grounded to earth: Don't these women know they are asking for trouble? No protection against the buildup of voltage.

The only position I've ever found relaxing in yoga is the final one, where I'm flat on my back on the floor and others start to snore. This is called the Corpse position. I'm nothing but ground.

V.

I turned fifty this year. I run on occasion and go to the gym to lift weights, but usually I walk. My favorite route circles Greenlake, which is next to the park where we used to run through the leaves on cross-country meets and is frequented by most of Seattle: you pass with an "On your left" or "On your right" warning. I walk there when I need to feel a sense of belonging, when I need to eat from the group dynamic. Greenlake is about watching and being watched. Greenlake is the kitchen where everyone gathers at the party because it's comfortable and it feels like home. I'm swept along in the current circling the lake. I'm part of the human race. I meet my friends there, and our focus is more social than sweat. We walk and talk, and we drink lattes afterwards and talk some more. An hour or two of therapy. That's my current version of gymnastics: verbal. Walking and talking at the same time. I'm a natural.

9

Gym Interrupted

Myrl Coulter

As a veteran of hundreds of workout classes, I have acquired a strange assortment of remnant clothing that lurks in the dark recesses of my closet: tiny shorts, striped tights, vicelike bra tops, and even leg warmers, all of which adorned my body at some time during the last twenty-five years. With such gym experience, you might expect that I've developed a female support network to sustain me during ups, downs, and in-betweens. Not exactly. Getting myself to the gym on a regular basis requires more fortitude, intestinal and otherwise, than I can consistently muster. After one of my prolonged absences, the prospect of stepping through that door again for the first time is daunting. All those tautly toned women who know how to speak the lingo, how to operate the equipment, and how to make their workouts look effortless do not rush to welcome newcomers or returnees. So I start, and then I stop, and eventually I start again.

The notion exists that women, or, to be more specific to my range of experience, middle-age, middle-class women in the northern regions of North America, support each other faithfully in all their endeavors, and thereby enjoy a great advantage over their already highly advantaged male counterparts, who struggle in stoic isolation, poor things.

At my gym, when I walk into a group class that has a token male or two in attendance, my focus is only momentarily diverted. Although they at times get more than their share of instructor attention, perhaps because the instructors in the classes I go to are almost always young and female, the men make no discernible dent in how the class session operates. The women just work around them, barely even acknowledging each other as they prepare to sweat.

Before a class begins, chatter is minimal; small smiles are shared only between veterans who have watched each other over a period of time and know where they fit in the fitness hierarchy. Emotionally revealing facial expressions are reserved for the actual working out part, and, even then, they can reveal only an intense desire to persevere through all the burning pain. I know that if I can't make it to the end of a set, there can be no change in my facial expression whatsoever. I also know that if I succeed and do make it across the set finish line, the same is required. In between sets, all female faces wear a calm, stoic mask designed to camouflage an inner dialogue that often sounds like this: Please don't make me do anything conspicuous. What's with all these mirrors? How does she do that? Omigod, she's got to be kidding. When this inner dialogue bursts through my calm exterior, I know that I am about to stop going to the gym again. The gym women will have to carry on without me.

Nevertheless, the gym women also draw me back. The last time I started again, it was because of a refreshing, longtime friend who lets her inner dialogue flow constantly and punctuates it with the most infectious laughter imaginable. After a particularly long absence during which I resigned myself to certain physical decay, my friend's refusal to give in to the old woman who was threatening to take over her body roused me from my physical stupor. Still, she had to bribe me: "Come to the gym with me and we'll have coffee afterwards." I don't even drink coffee anymore, but the promise of an hour's conversation with a fine friend was more than enough to send me digging through my stored old clothes for a pair of tights. Fortunately, I left the leg warmers behind.

Also fortunately, I have long since lost track of the high school gym uniform that my schoolmates and I had to wear: a crisp (I even had to iron it) white cotton shirt—with a collar and buttons no less—and navy blue short shorts with built-in bloomers to conceal any stray underwear that might inadvertently be exposed during the distinctly "un-ladylike" (to quote my mother, grandmother, or any aunt who happened to be around) poses we were about to throw our bodies into. The thought of that ridiculous uniform instantly brings to mind an image of my much younger self going from station to station in my high school gym doing push-ups and jumping jacks and other impossible calisthenics while listening to the boys on the opposite side of the partitioned gym playing a rousing game of something that produced great guffaws of laughter on their side and insatiable curiosity on ours. After high school, my gym experiences would be interrupted for several years as I got down to the business of finding a husband, and a job to keep me occupied while I did so, activities my family and countless others expected of young women newly graduated from high school in 1968.

I can't remember what I wore five or so years later when, now safely a married woman living far away from both high school and family, I went to a yoga class with a newfound friend one cold winter night. This session was very unlike the yoga classes offered at today's trendy studios. Current yoga enthusiasts, sleek in their trim low-slung pants and matching tops made out of magic technical fabrics that not only work with every movement but also somehow seem to assist in the completion of those movements, float into beautiful rooms that have soothing music playing softly in the background, exotic incense tantalizing the nostrils, and glowing tealights softly illuminating a warm hardwood floor. No, my first yoga class was in a gym on a military base on the East Coast. The only "music" came from the beat of the basketball game going on in the next gym; the only scent was of disinfectant and forgotten smelly socks lost under the bleachers somewhere; and the harsh glare from the mercury vapor lights far up in the rafters did not softly illuminate anything. That night I learned that my yoga capabilities were far from a natural talent, and that any progress I made in achieving a fluid facility for the practice would be hard earned.

Afterwards, in the locker room, while everyone was changing from exercise clothing back into the bulky warm gear required to venture outside, my friend glanced around the room at our female classmates now in various states of undress. Covertly she leaned over and whispered into my ear: "There really are no perfect bodies, are there?" This remark stays with me as a kind of awakening, a moment of realization that women not only put themselves up against an impossible standard, but they also hold the women around them up (or down) to that standard as well. It would take me many more years to begin to dissect that impossible standard and the roots of its existence, but for that moment in my still-young life, it did give me pause. My friend and I would become very close for that short period: military life makes for intense, fast friendships that can be severed from their regimented moorings at any moment. Like my relationship with gyms across the land, our closeness has been interrupted regularly over the years.

The next interruption to my gym life came courtesy of motherhood. Having three children in two years (the second one turned out to be twins) meant that I really didn't have to think much about fitness. In fact, I really didn't have time to think much about anything.

In the two years after my twins were born, only one world event remains vivid in my mind: Elvis died one August day and I cried for my lost youth and freedom. During the years that my children were of preschool age, I occasionally found time to play racquetball with a friend. Also a mother of twins, she was better at the game than I was, but I didn't care. All I wanted to do was beat the hell out of that ball for an hour or so, preferably on a court where no one could see us, and then retreat to the nearest bar for a glass of wine. It was a night out. I didn't care about what I looked like or what I wore; in fact, I considered myself lucky to rummage around in a laundry basket and find something that was both mine and clean, much less stylish.

Eventually, however, the urge to sweat returned. I joined a suburban gym so as to work a few aerobics classes into a schedule that, at the time, included a full-time job and three children in elementary school. These were the days of skinny striped headbands, funky leg warmers, and matching body suits. Of throbbing loud music and that plague of aerobics fanatics—shin splints. We loved our slim, bouncy instructor who made our workouts more like dance routines, who shouted happily at us that we could do it, we could make it, we could shake it. Ours was a group that came together for exercise but somehow bonded in a way that the shared coffees afterwards were equally important. Soon we even gathered together for entirely social evenings, bringing mates, appetizers, and common concerns about our kids. Having had a few personal disruptions in my life, a divorce, and a new marriage, this group was a welcome oasis of social conventionality in my life. Less about fitness and more about community, individual body dynamics didn't seem to matter.

Gradually, the appeal of my aerobics period waned as some of the group members drifted on to other things. Soon the pressures on my time became increasingly difficult to manage, and the suburban gym was off my regular travel path. Inevitably, I stopped going. I punctuated this interruption in my gym life with the occasional effort to venture outside and establish a running routine for myself. I would sporadically head out down into the wondrous river valley that characterizes my city, guiltily leaving my dog at home because the park was off limits to her, and my running feet always took me in the direction of that park. Despite living in a body that clearly wasn't built for running—short legs, low center of gravity, bottom heavy—I surprised myself by being able to bring an endurance to the activity I didn't know I had. This endurance helped make up for the fact that I'm probably among the slowest runners ever to lace up a far-too-expensive new pair of trainers. I envisioned myself as a human version of the energizer bunny stuck on low speed. My running career didn't last, but not because I didn't enjoy running; I did. I often felt the solitude was the best part of it, but the solitude also got in my way. Nobody expected me to show up, and nobody urged me to carry on. In the end, only I noticed when I stopped doing it. I did, however, end up with unique fresh additions to my wardrobe: running tights, wind jackets, baseball caps, and several pairs of running shoes, one that even had an air pump in each heel.

After making a few halfhearted efforts to get involved in other fitness activities at our local YMCA, I soon just stopped making any attempts at physical fitness whatsoever. Interrupted again, I simply ignored my body and avoided gyms entirely for a few years. I worked, socialized, raised my teenagers, and convinced myself that walking the dog would take care of any exercise I needed. Unsurprisingly, my fitness level deteriorated at a rate directly proportional to the larger clothing sizes I needed. One year during this period, my husband bought me a treadmill for Christmas. It was well used for a while, mostly by my daughters, but, like bodies, it needed maintenance. Too often. During prolonged times of disrepair, it stood idle. When I thought it had begun to glare at me, I just closed the door.

Facing an empty house after the three young adults all moved out at around the same time, I decided to simplify our lives and clear out some clutter. I sold the treadmill to my sister-in-law and finally admitted I needed to join a gym again. Or, rather, a "fitness center." Gyms had been renamed, but that wasn't all. I was surprised to find that a fitness center revolution had taken place while I wasn't paying attention. The first thing I noticed was the equipment: everywhere I looked I saw cardio machines, racks of dumbbells and free weights, fitness balls, and a plethora of strange-looking devices with pulleys and attachments. I had to search to find a room that even resembled my obviously outdated idea of what a gymnasium used to be. Finally, there it was, off in a corner, a downsized room, elegantly labeled a "studio," that played host to classes with odd-sounding new names: step, spinning, pilates. A whole new gym world existed, and I had missed its genesis.

Strange equipment and a multitude of weight machines weren't the only new things at the gym. Cool, toned, athletic bodies were everywhere. Personal trainers led their charges through structured routines, feeding them into the equipment like dough into a pasta machine: plump and shapeless on entry, hopefully coming out lean and flat at the other end. Rows of treadmills sat beside more rows of stair climbers and cross-trainers; the still-present stationary bicycles looked almost archaic beside the new models of cardiac training devices. Some gym goers seemed to spend hours on a treadmill, only to get off and step immediately onto a cross-trainer for another hour. Water bottles and personal music devices were the new accessory requirements. Televisions hung from the ceilings, placed at convenient angles so that everywhere an eye looked it could have visual distraction. News, soap operas, weather, sports, talk shows, and music videos—all the banalities of Western society's rampant consumer culture had entered the gym experience. As one who is both repelled by and attracted to popular culture, I hesitated to accept this addition as a positive one.

Nevertheless, I was back. I bought in. After a few months of regular attendance on my own, I decided to challenge myself. Perhaps it was loneliness, perhaps it was curiosity, or maybe just because I could. Anyway, for whatever reason, I decided to try working with a personal trainer. I was assigned to a charming young woman. She assessed my body very scientifically, fat mass and all, tested me out on a few weight machines, talked to me about nutrition and the need for regular workouts, the whole package. We set up a schedule: once a week I worked out with her, the rest of the week on my own. To my surprise I took to this new regimen. I liked the balance, the expectation that every seven days I would work out with someone I could talk to and who could tell me how I was doing, and also the expectation that each week I would come to her having worked out regularly since our last meeting. Things went along well for several months.

During this time, I was largely oblivious to what went on at the gym. I didn't really pay attention to who was working out when, who was wearing what, or even to what I was wearing. I found myself the most nondescript comfort clothing possible, deciding not to enter the fashion arena that the gym seemed to have become. Single-minded focus was my new mandate. As it turned out, I was oblivious even to the obvious. My lovely personal trainer had to draw my attention to her emerging condition: she was pregnant and would be taking an extended maternity leave soon. Outwardly, I gave the expected response—a squeal, a hug, motherly reminiscences of the joys to come. Inwardly, I was churlish: What about me? How could you do this to me? We have a system going, and you're going to leave me? In retrospect, I like to think that my reaction was a little less self-absorbed than that, and beneath my dismay, I truly was happy for her. Ever gracious, she assured me that I could do it on my own, and that if I didn't want to wait for her return, she'd be happy to recommend one of the other trainers around the club. I said I would be fine. A few months later, my personal trainer had a healthy baby boy and all the gym people, myself included, helped celebrate his arrival. After the excitement of the birth died down, I went to the gym exactly twice. Six months later, I cancelled my membership. Gym interrupted, again.

For the next few years, I fell into my old habit of avoiding fitness of any kind. To my great good fortune, at this low physical point, my fabulous friend with the infectious laugh returned to my life's sphere. She and her struggle with the old woman who wanted her body gave me renewed incentive: someone expected me to walk through that gym door. Or, rather, the "health club" door, fitness centers-cum-gyms having gained another new moniker during my recent sojourn away. Happily, my aging body responded positively. I liked the reunion with the machines, the regular routine, the chats while on the bikes or the treadmills, the challenges we threw out to each other, like balancing on the fitness ball until we fell off amid peals of laughter, disrupting the normally stoic atmosphere, and getting some disapproving looks in the process. I was back. I was a gym person once more. Soon I booked a few sessions with a new personal trainer to add more depth to my newest program. Living life in this body was good again.

In between balancing on balls and laughing with my funny friend, I looked around my new "health club." In my absence, things had changed again. For a while I couldn't really figure out what it was, but I soon came to a surprising realization. It wasn't the physical environs that had changed this time but the people. Gym people now came in all shapes and ages. Old and young, big and small, male and female all circulated in, on, and around the equipment, taking turns, sometimes nodding and friendly, sometimes cool and remote. And on many of these varied bodies, a new physical feature was notable: cleavage, strikingly set off by fashionable new gym attire, which suited the young, the trim, and the voluptuous. The always confusing, at least to me, North American obsession with the female breast seemed to be at an all time high and driven by the owners of the breasts themselves. Many gym women appeared to have fallen in love with their upper body attributes and proudly presented them for the gym world's viewing pleasure. At times, I found myself watching, fascinated by the shapely young women preparing for their workouts in the locker room, posing, puckering, and positioning their parts in front of the mirror for long minutes before making an entrance into the public arena. After they left I would sometimes glance at my own reflection, but mine was a perfunctory look. No need for me to position anything.

I was enjoying a bright glorious gym time, but, predictably, yet another interruption was just around the corner. One day my fabulous friend moved away. After she left, I kept going, but I couldn't stop myself from looking for her whenever I was there. I went less often: I didn't immediately abandon my schedule, but nevertheless, my visits dwindled and soon came to a complete halt again. Months of malaise passed until, one day, my phone rang. The voice on the other end was that of the personal trainer with whom I had worked so briefly. What's happening? Where are you? Come back, she said. I couldn't really think of a good reason not to, and she was so very nice to have called, so I did.

And that's where things stand now. We've mapped out a new schedule, one that, so far, works for me. I've even added to my gym wardrobe, replacing my anonymous T-shirts and ill-fitting shorts with a few pairs of "active"-wear pants made of smooth technical fabric that I like to think makes me look like a gym girl and maybe even helps me move a little. I drew the line at those cleavage-producing bra tops, however, after spending an afternoon in a store dressing room trying to find a reasonable way to get in or out of one of those things. That's a workout in itself. Somewhat appropriately attired, I'm back in gym mode; this time around, it's contemplative mode, somewhat solitary and, dare I say it, mature. While my body works up a sweat, my brain uses the time to muse over whatever happens to be floating around in it. Treadmill time, it turns out, is good thinking time.

For those of us fortunate enough to live in able bodies we can take to the gym, and for those of us fortunate enough that we don't have to spend every minute of our days scraping for basic survival needs or struggling against overt oppression, life is full of choices. Life is also a series of interruptions. People we love and people we just like a lot come into our lives, but also go out again. We take jobs, and we leave them. We start new endeavors and abandon old ones. The one relationship we have that isn't interrupted, at least until the day it permanently ends, is the one we have with our bodies. The most intimate connection we have to our time on this planet, our bodies are home to the lives we live, and the lives we live show on them.

Looking around the gym today, I realize that my old friend from that yoga class long ago might have to admit that these days there are some "perfect" bodies roaming through these busy health club locker rooms. The male physiques that populate the gym are often breathtaking in bulk, astonishing in their musculature and tone. However, appreciative as I am of a well-maintained male body, it's often the female bodies that draw my attention. When I see young women with incredibly slim hips and impossibly large breasts, I am at first puzzled that this version of so-called physical perfection in fact exists and then perplexed at anyone's need to fulfill this artificial requirement.

For me, the most intriguing bodies are all the others. The bodies that have distinctly "unperfect" shapes, the bodies that show they carry stories with them, the lived-in bodies that don't deny their accumulated experiences—both positive and negative—are the ones that most eloquently bear witness to life's many contingencies and interruptions.

10

Naked Truth

Lynn Z. Bloom

Bounding into the Mansfield Community Center on a bright sunny Saturday, my loaded gym bag banging into my leg, I ran into David, a physics professor, retired for a decade. He seems softer, more subdued in recent weeks, since Carolanne, his wife, died of cancer at age fifty-nine in mid-July. We exchanged the usual "Hello." "Nice day." "How are you?" "Fine," aware of Carolanne's almost palpable presence, unspoken. For this is where we all used to hang out together, David and Carolanne, Martin and I, talking regularly over coffee in the lobby, conversations that became more specific when Carolanne and I left for the women's locker room. My aim was always to exercise hard enough to break into a T-shirt soaking sweat like hers, even at the risk of growing as weary as she sometimes looked. But swimmers, especially those as inept as I, don't sweat.

Though Carolanne modestly discounted her strength, agility, and daring, it was clear that her resolute commitment to exercise and her fierce energy were the driving forces behind the couple's worldwide wilderness explorations. She had hiked in Peru, three miles high, and in Chilean Patagonia; filmed king penguins eye to eye in the muddy Falklands; trekked New Zealand's Milford Track (more mud!); and photographed—this time for National Geographic's *Adventure* magazine—a river rafting trip in the Burnside River area of the Arctic Circle. The other women and I marveled over her accounts of extraordinary exploits, invariably understated. So when she attributed a pain in her side to fatigue from portaging a kayak and sixty-five pounds of photographic gear long distances in the Canadian Territories, that seemed reasonable, despite the fact that she still seemed extraordinarily fit. Who wouldn't be tired? But by Thanksgiving, when the fatigue dragged on, and the pain kicked in, the diagnosis was colon cancer. On rare good days, she would show up at the Rec Center, long bob glowing (I later realized it was a wig), resolute and resilient. The last time I saw her was in the locker room, after we'd had to uninvite her and David to dinner because I had a cold that could have sent her compromised immune system into a steep decline.

Summer Trips

In most social contexts, when asked "How are you?" we automatically reply "Fine." I could have told David "I'm facing a third rotator cuff surgery," but I chose not to. But in the locker room it's different, because we're naked, and there's no place to hide—except in the toilet stalls, where only the modest teenage girls go to change, out of thong underwear into bikini bathing suits. For over thirty years I have swum laps every day, sometimes varied with fast walking and more recently with strengthening exercises. What began in hopes of preventing the family heritage of arthritis (so far, so good, knock wood) has become a way of life. On dreary, draggy days when even grading papers seems like a welcome alternative to slogging through heavy weather to the gym, I think of the doctor's office cartoon, "What can't you work into your schedule? A half hour of exercise, or twenty-four hours of being dead?" and I'm out of the house like a shot.

However, no good deed goes unpunished. Five years ago the decades of swimming resulted in a torn right rotator cuff that had to be repaired. The punishment was exacerbated when aggressive physical therapy exercises ripped out the pin and all the stitches—my jock doc orthopedist and his staff calibrate the rehab to the age and agility of the UConn athletes they treat rather than gearing it down for their less resilient clientele—and I needed a second surgery to redo the first. There went my hope of healing up faster than anyone on this planet. This time it's the left shoulder, an injury that came after sailing full speed ahead through the summer abroad, embedded in an ironic crash landing in August, at home.

Last summer, when I was teaching creative writing in Florence for six weeks, Martin and I walked happily over every kilometer of this city, bellissimo, four to six hours a day. In addition, we had to climb a total of several hundred steps to our apartment, a block from the Duomo, and my classroom and the faculty office in the Palazzo Rucellai. After Florence, we hiked for two weeks in the Swiss Alps with our children and adolescent grandchildren, every day encountering a mixture of rain, hail, sleet, snow, and occasional sunshine. No problems, not a slip, trip, or single sore muscle.

But at home in Connecticut, walking at my usual brisk pace to attend a jazz benefit for the local hospital's emergency room a few hours after Carolanne's memorial service, I caught my foot in a wire stretched over the concrete sidewalk, fell flat on my nose, chin, shoulders, knuckles, and knees. I spent the evening in the ER; no broken bones, not even a rip in my slacks. Several weeks of persistent pain later, however, an MRI revealed a big tear in the left rotator cuff.

I share this information only with pals at the gym, and then only selectively. No one else wants to hear even this six-sentence recitation, though my knee-jerk reaction is to tell the truth. So when a friend at the theater asked "How are you?" I began, "I'm facing a third rotator cuff surgery . . ." before her out-of-focus look signaled that all she really wanted to hear was "Fine." So I trailed off, "But really, I'm fine." "That's good," she said, and turned back to her program.

At Work and at Play in the Gym

The Widow. Until the surgery with its anticipated four-to-six months of postop PT, I can continue swimming if I use only the breaststroke or sidestroke. Not a problem. A new swimmer appears, a woman so attractive, her radiant white hair forming such a luminous halo as she traverses the lane next to mine, that I am impelled to talk to her. "Welcome," I say, recognizing on her wrist the plastic tape given to people with a one-day pass. As we navigate the lanes, up and down, the conversation begins with the neutral, "My friend"—she gesticulates toward a much younger woman in the warm therapy pool—"brought me here. It's a nice pool." The Community Center pool is indeed a nice, clean, new, well-lighted place open from 5 a.m. to 10 p.m.; the coffee's on until noon in the airy lounge, equipped with Internet, large-screen TV, magazines, and board books for bored toddlers. "It's good to get out," she offers after a few laps. "My husband died four months ago." "Oh, how sad," I say, but she smiles, "He had Alzheimer's for ten years, but he was only in hospice care for a couple of weeks." "What a tough time," I reply with deliberate ambiguity. "Did you have any relief?" "A couple of weeks a year a respite caregiver came in so I could get some time away. Other than that I was with him 24/7, all day every day. I could never leave."

Without a shred of self-pity, during lap upon lap she lays out the routine, hour by hour, day after day. Finally she beams, "It's so good to be in this water," a welcome baptism indeed. Flirtatious eyes scan the other lanes. "I'd like to meet a new man, do you know any?" I don't even know her, though I now know her life. "What about a club or an organization you like—Audubon hikes, Habitat for Humanity, book discussions, the Covenant Soup Kitchen"—these may say more about my interests than about hers. "That way you could have something enjoyable to do, whether or not you meet someone to date." "Date?" she laughs, "I'd really like to get married again." "And I'd like to see you again," she says as we return to the locker room. "My pleasure," I reply.

The Cyclist. I don't tell my new acquaintance about the impending rotator cuff repair, but I do bring it up with another locker-room long-timer, a librarian with a young daughter and a big, happy dog I've passed on my way home. "Oh," she says on hearing the news, "I tore the meniscus in my knee when I fell off my bike in July, and I'm having surgery November 6. Who's your doctor?" The same as mine. We'll try to schedule PT at the same time, same rehab center near campus. Both of us expect to be back at work within a day or two after the oxymoronically named "outpatient surgery," as if the bloody deed were to be performed in the hospital parking lot, or possibly outsourced to Bangalore.

The Survivor. In the locker room three weeks ago I encountered another friend—a high-level university administrator, now retired—a fast-walking gym regular whom I hadn't seen all summer, erect, slender, poised as usual. Her foot was in a cast. "What happened?" I ask. "I broke it," she says." "Doing what?" "Walking, just walking in a shopping mall." "How is that possible?" With a grimace she replied, "Osteoporosis. My doctor says my bones are so fragile that they could break even while I'm sitting down. I'm not supposed to drive, but I live alone and I can't go anywhere without driving." She added, "While you were in Italy they discovered breast cancer. I've had a lumpectomy and radiation." All around us the high school girls' swimming team was changing clothes, lamenting heartbreak and weight gain, oblivious to our conversation. "Oh, no!" I groaned, and when she said, "At the three-month checkup the doctor said it's in the nodes in the other breast," I offered a speechless hug, future help—and decided to skip the rotator cuff information.

I did not see her again until today when from the lap lane I spied her in the therapy pool. There she was, looking blonder and better than ever; what had happened? The hardness in the nodes, she said, was caused by an infection, not the spread of cancer; she had just gotten the results. "I'm celebrating," she rejoiced. "My former college roommate is coming to visit. I'm marinating a pork roast, I've made a chocolate torte, and bought a good bottle of wine." The girls' swimming team, attracted by the menu, snaps to eavesdropping alertness. "Now I can call myself a 'cancer survivor.' " I realize how rarely we discuss food in the locker room, and how welcome is this verbal feast. I tell her, "You're the only person I know who, even when naked, looks as if she's dressed for cocktails." The locker room erupts in laughter, "I accept the award! I accept!" she exults, and prances out as if I'd just given her an Oscar, her cast still on.

The Real Athletes. I have never been able to pitch, bat, throw, pass, shoot, or hit a ball; the orthopedist tells me my "loose joints" are responsible for this ineptitude as well as for the rotator cuff injury. For that matter, I can't run or swim either with any accuracy, speed, or distance, and I attribute this to genes, not joints. Year after year, I have never gotten any better—but athletic improvement has never, for me, been the point. So I never compare myself to the people at the gym whom I consider the real athletes, a cool, elegant crew with taut bodies, tight lips. The Masters Swimmers, tearing up and down the lanes for ninety minutes at a time, two of them consistent winners in the Senior Olympics. The marathon competitors and the triathletes, risking their spandexed lives daily to get to the gym via predawn cycling on Connecticut's narrow, winding roads with no shoulders. The horse trainer, whose sexy underwear counterpoints her Speedo swimsuit and no-nonsense jeans, never jodhpurs. Carolanne, her red parka a vivid slash among the snowy peaks of Patagonia. What would be the point?

The Swimmers' Table

At Carolanne's memorial lunch, hosted by David with amazing grace, I was pleased to be included at the swimmers' table. There we were. A Masters Swimmer, himself facing a rotator cuff operation as a consequence of all that good exercise. A friend with MS who, although she needs a wheelchair for land locomotion, has in the past year increased her swimming endurance from one-half to sixteen laps—a mile, says "I'd live in the pool all day if I could." Her physical therapist is also at the table, as are another determined regular and her husband, both Holocaust survivors, whose round-the-world flight (Amsterdam, Vienna, London, Melbourne) ended with their arrival in Connecticut via a post-World War II immigration quota. The most elegant of us all is a pretty, petite woman who cheerfully reminds me that two years ago, after she'd told me she was newly widowed, I said, "You look as if you need a hug," and gave her one. It is strange to see these veterans of the deep, of life itself, dressed up, in homage to Carolanne. It is strange to see them dressed at all—scars, sags, splints—evidence of mortality we take for granted in the locker room now covered up. We joke about our appearance, as we do when meeting at concerts, plays, the grocery store, university receptions, anywhere but the gym, "I can hardly recognize you with clothes on." We know each other naked. We know the naked truth, and that truth has set us free, to live as we will die, with every fiber of body and of mind.

11

Women's Yoga

A Multigenre Meditation on Language and the Body

Victoria Boynton

On a good day, the yoga studio is a thoughtless place, a space where thought falls away, leaving a mindless body—a relief, a surprise, a miracle, really. Yoga practitioners cultivate this miraculous mindlessness in the bubble of the yoga studio—a space that acts as a container in which to experience this mindless body. Ordinarily, as busy women in a busy world, our busy minds ignore the body. Yoga allows us to pay attention to our bodies as we let go of our mental chatter. Medical research on the benefits of yoga and meditation shows that the temporary surrender of the mind through the ancient practices of yoga and meditation can prove to be powerful survival strategies for anyone, but especially for women. As women continue to step into positions of power and as expectations of women increase, women will need practices, spaces, and communities devoted to detaching from the everyday mind with all of its compulsions, stresses, and strivings.

For millennial professional women, the yoga studio is a luxurious support. When the mind lets go, the deep relaxation that results nourishes the body and soothes the care-worn identity. When women enter the thoughtless space of the yoga studio, they are encouraged to lay themselves out, to loosen and surrender to the body's presence—a presence that is ultimately shifting, undeniably fluid, and basically unrepresentable because it is beyond language.

The protected space of the studio encourages the yoga practitioner to let go of the defense mechanisms and psychic armor that she habitually must employ to operate powerfully in the outside world. As that outside world falls away, she begins to inhabit her body as a space beyond language, an open, breathing space. The presence of other women doing the same thing increases the power of the practice. This collective exercise promotes an intense experience of the body, its morphing physicality, its slippery identity, temporary as the breath itself.

Preparation

> Lay out a mat,
> fingers, breasts,
> feet, face, lay out
> the eager gravity of age
> the lax coccyx
> the feral love-handle
> and the troubling.
> Lay out the strait-laced
> backbone and the sacred
> bone of sacrifice,
> fused at the spine's end,
> and lay out the jawbone,
> tight as a trap. Lay out
> the magic coxa and
> the pelvic bowl, cup of hip,
> and fine lined skin. Lay out
> the being and trying to be.
> Lay it all out;
> your mat is an alter.
> Then leave.
> Your body will wait for the gods
> to start tinkering with
> these abandoned offerings.

Postmodern theory has powerfully interrogated identity and the body, arguing a radical instability of the body that reminds me strongly of the results of yoga and meditation practice. In a yoga class, my experience of the mindless body parallels the descriptions of postmodern subjects as unstable and non-unitary. The identities of subjects are constructed in multiple and contradictory processes of becoming.

Though there is no definable, solid being at the center of identity, there is a welter of moment-to-moment experience, infinitely complex and shifting. Yoga practitioners in the midst of practice often experience their identity as fluid and contradictory: through their intense physical engagement with and attention to the body, it seems both to be hyperpresent and to disappear. A revolutionary presence results—a sort of slipping out of identity (a stilling of distracting mentality and habitual discourses) as the body comes into focus, suddenly central to existence in the moment.

All We Are Is

In fact
all we are is
one heartbeat
one breath
one bloody rush
of pulse.
Now, all we are is.

This version of the body is in striking contrast to the social construction of the normative, material body in the world, a construction that encourages an obsessive striving to match unattainable models alternately governed by norms of beauty, business, social, political, and economic power. So to enter another space in which a woman is encouraged to relax out of these tight fits is to enter a sacred space, that is, a space that points to and loosens women's allegiance to the oppressive social.

The studios themselves work on their practitioners. For instance, Wendy Sagar's studio in Truth or Consequences, New Mexico, is full of beautiful things, artfully arranged. What a pleasure this studio space is with its incense, its bronze Buddha and Ganesh, its subtle prayer rugs and bright Mexican hangings. We women in the class gather, leaving a pile of shoes at the door, lay mats and blankets and props on the polished wood floor, creating our own narrow spaces, one for each body—a grounding container for letting go of our incessant thinking and finding the body in the present moment. We each create our own space capsule, separate and private as well as connected to all the other spaces occupied by all the other women: separation and connection at once. Jai Hari's studio space, in a beautifully rehabilitated house in downtown Ithaca, New York, is comparatively simple, its empty beauty a supporting presence in its own way. Even the big exercise room at the Ithaca YMCA is transformed by yoga instructor Mo Viele as she leads her large classes into quiet attention to the body. But whatever studio space or teacher, the safety, calm, and encouragement to pay attention work powerful, connective magic. The studio is a respite from busy-ness, a constructed space apart from the business of thinking, doing, having. It is an undoing place, a place beyond the words, sentences, and automatic thinking that governs our ordinary experience. The hyper-consciousness of our bodies in the contained studio gives language a different spin. The teacher's instructions begin to sound like a chant, and as we move into the class, most of what she expresses is communicated nonverbally. Language leaks away, leaving us with an unfamiliar, momentary clarity.

We may do yoga by ourselves at home, but being in the yoga studio and having a teacher who guides us allows a kind of relaxation unavailable when we are directing our own practice on our living room floors. Someone else speaks simple instructions; we listen, and our bodies respond in remarkable ways. It is the body, surely, the body in all its gendered and aged particularity, and yet a question arises: What is the body? As we do yoga, we are paradoxically hyper-aware of our bodies, of the rising and falling lungs, for instance. We become conscious of the body, from head to toe—we know each part and yet, paradoxically, yoga practice breaks down the body so that it becomes not a sum of constituent parts but a process, not a concrete thing but a blur of motion and shift. The body-as-thing falls apart as we experience it in process rather than as object.

This breakdown of the body parallels the way language breaks down during a yoga session or in meditation or at various other times when signifiers slip, terms lose their foundations, and denotation detonates, words fragmenting and flying everywhere. At these times, there is an opening beyond what we expect and beyond what we can articulate in sentences.

Yoga Ocean Breath

Breathing, you are a sea of light, warm slosh of creature
netted into herself, touching her wavy becoming.
You: dissolve,
your memory, your habit,
that tyranny of sentences familiar as an echo become only
rising and falling tide, yourself only breath,
each shining cell an ocean-moon call,

flesh pulled, tucked around your bed of bone
stone shining marrow dance—even this rock of
ribs, pelvis, spine, skull holds swift water.

Breath the belly balloon, rubber band diaphragm,
lung top tipping the cup of breath up into your throat,
heart hugging breath, electric spray of you—all
the way down through shoulder, bicep sinew,
simmering elbow to wrist, palm, finger. Ocean breath:
waves open you, flume through your breast, flood
through your brain like sun, ocean in a gland,
your scalp a sea, your face an infinity.
Lean your cheek on your hand.
Breathe down the fall of hip/thigh/knee/calf/shin/ankle/heel/
    sole/toe
the foam of it, the swirl.
Spirals through neck back butt, back up to lung and out,
each pore a heart, a sea of light.

As we stretch, the restless twitter of the mind dissolves. All we hear
is the ocean breath of the woman next to us and feel her sea of light
expand. We join—human chain. The experience convinces us that we
are not separate. Listen, here are words for who you are:

At the Yoga Studio

"Do nothing" say the teachers.
You lie like a corpse,
obey the instruction—breath, breath—
clearing you, cell by cell,
until after a while,
you're see-through
watery, airy
somewhere where metaphor
is a ladder rung, thin as a hair
you're climbing
(up or down?)
on nothing
thinking,
"It's stupid to write poems
about yoga."

"Right," you reply.
But the *R* in *Right*
is coming apart and the *i* too and even
the *gh*, ordinarily inseparable,
separate—
noiselessly *g* goes down
swishing its fishy tail,
while *h* flies up, out of sight
with the kite of *t* . . . "Where am I?"
you think. The notes of your voice,
lost, float by, down through
layers of water
into a dark where illuminated
fish make light of themselves.
Light comes apart,
the *L*, the *i*, the *gh* again,
again the *t* floats away.
You climb out of your mind
into your body, your white
heartbeat rising
through the dark,
with the enormity of
an old cliche,
to meet you.

Within the yoga studio, women can shuck the concretions of the mind and in that radical, momentary transformation form a powerful connection with each other. The intimacy of the studio's silence speaks its own language of community.

Part 3

■

On the Road, the Slopes, and the Lake

12

"Messing about in Boats"

Rowing as *l'Écriture Féminine*

Shannon Smith

In Kenneth Grahame's Edwardian children's novel *The Wind in the Willows* (1933 [1908]), the self-assured character Rat sings the praises of sculling to his riverbank friend Mole: "Believe me, my young friend, there is *nothing*—absolutely nothing—half so much worth doing as simply messing about in boats" (8, emphasis in original). For Rat, rowing on the river provides a momentary escape from the day-to-day realities of animal life. The pair of sculls in his hand, cutting through the water, expresses the freedom from obligation that the practice of rowing entails for the "joyous oarsman" (8). Rowing for Rat is an outward movement, free from the linear constraints of an origin and a destination: "Whether you get away, or whether you don't; whether you arrive at your destination or whether you reach somewhere else. . . . Nothing seems to really matter, that's the charm of it" (8). A similar freeing act of expression is described by Hélène Cixous in the 1975 essay "The Laugh of the Medusa" in which she discusses the textual practice of *l'écriture féminine*, a mode of creative expression that contrasts with the standard model of "male writing" that is inextricably "confounded with the history of reason" (2001 [1975], 2042–43).

I have always thought that rowing is much like writing. The movement of the oar through the water is the expression of that which exists on the edge of a rower's conscious mind—perhaps thoughts deemed inappropriate for expression off the water, desires thick and fluid as the medium through which the oar moves. I have always thought that these expressions in the water are creative. As the blade of the oar moves through the water, forming puddles—giant thumbprints, round curves ending in a smirk of playful, white foam—momentum is created that smoothly propels the rower forward. The movement of the body during a strong stroke is like liquid; the concentric circles left behind in the water are, to those who choose to read, a text that can reveal much about the individual rower who writes it as well as the state of the crew of which she is a part. This text has a motion of its own, soon returning to the watery subconscious from which it was first formed, but it bears the contributions of a community of rowers, all of whom participate in its writing.

This understanding of the communal creative potential of the stroke of an oar is not one that fits with the traditional cultural understanding of the sport of rowing. At the center of boathouse culture is the figure of the manly rower, a mythic construction that draws attention to the characteristics of strength (both physical and mental), endurance, and an aggressive, competitive mentality that harkens back to the sport's ancient martial origins. Scholars of sport such as Varda Burstyn have identified such a culture as inherently masculinist in that it is "both about and supportive of men's gender dominance" through participation in the sport (Burstyn 1998, 10). It is a culture perhaps best exemplified by memoirs of the sport, such as Daniel Topolski's (1989) account of the turbulent 1986–1987 racing season at the Oxford University Boat Club (OUBC), *True Blue: The Oxford Boat Race Mutiny*. Though in this setting a sense of community among members of a crew is cultivated, nothing is as valuable as the individual oarsman. This is exemplified in Topolski's description of the OUBC's president, Donald Macdonald: "Donald would drive his sculling boat through mile after mile, in a silent brutal programme of conditioning—he would work all along, at first light, punishing himself without mercy. His was the private dignity of the lone athlete, with a grim purpose, fighting a solitary war with himself, towards a goal only he can see" (51). In the economy of this culture, wielding an oar is not creative but rather controlling. The "grim purpose" of "conditioning" and "punishing" is not a generative expression of the inner life of the rower but rather a "silent" and "solitary war" that is fought, and won, alone. The water becomes not a surface and a source for the text but an enemy to be scarred and subdued.

Though Cixous states that "it is impossible to *define* a feminine practice of writing" because the desire to define belongs to the controlling impulses of the "discourse that regulates the phallocentric system" (2001 [1975], 2046, emphasis in original), it is possible to reach an understanding of *l'écriture féminine* that will aid in locating this mode of expression in other cultural practices; more specifically, a summary of the major concepts that make up *l'écriture féminine* will help demonstrate the affinity between Cixous's idea of writing "women's imaginary" (2040) and the cultural practice I have called "messing about in boats," or rowing as a woman.

Though *l'écriture féminine* is best understood as a linguistic expression of all that has been associated with "woman" and dubbed Other in a masculinist culture, Cixous does not intend for the practice of *l'écriture féminine* to be limited to the act of writing but rather opened up to include all manners of expression, including speech, song, and artistic work. *L'écriture féminine* is a practice of reclamation and redefinition, its purpose "to break up, to destroy; and to foresee the unforeseeable, to project" (2040). As a means of maintaining the balance of power in a masculinist or phallocentric culture, woman, and thus all that her body signifies, is labeled a "Dark Continent" and taught to fear this Othered potential: "As soon as [women] begin to speak, at the same time as they're taught their name, they can be taught that their territory is black. . . . Dark is dangerous. You can't see anything in the dark. . . . And so we have internalized this horror of the dark" (2041). In writing "women's imaginary" (2040), one is not simply reversing the gender binary but moving beyond it. It is this idea of motion that is central to Cixous's understanding of the way in which women can move beyond the idea of "man/woman" and thus insert themselves "into the text—as into the world and into history" (2039). Abigail Bray, in her discussion of some of Cixous's major concepts, chooses to understand this movement as a distinguishing feature of Cixous's "female libidinal economy—an economy of desire which is open, productive [and] creative" (Bray 2004, 52). Woman moves in this economy through the practice of *l'écriture féminine* and thus is able to express the "subversive, dissident energy which is capable of transforming metaphysics, language, [and] social relations" (56). As Cixous states:

> Her writing can only keep going, without ever inscribing or discerning contours, daring to make these vertiginous crossings of the other(s) ephemeral and passionate sojourns in him, her, them, whom she inhabits long enough to look at from the point closest to their drives, and then further, impregnated through and through with these brief identificatory embraces, she goes and passes into infinity. (2001 [1975], 2052)

This mode of expression that "can only keep going, without ever inscribing or discerning contours" (2052) is also found in the practice of rowing as a woman, especially as it is described by Sara Hall in her 2002 memoir *Drawn to the Rhythm: A Passionate Life Reclaimed*. Through examining the ways in which Hall's understanding of her rowing practice echoes Cixous's elaboration of the practice and effects of *l'écriture féminine*, I argue that the practice of rowing as a woman is another manner of expression that can be included with those artistic, linguistic, and musical that Cixous suggests are part of this *"new insurgent* writing which . . . will allow [woman] to carry out the indispensable ruptures and transformations in her history" (2001 [1975], 2043, emphasis in original). One of the products of this specific practice of *l'écriture féminine* is a bodily community that is characterized by its open economy. Cixous describes this economy as "body with out end, without appendage, without principal "parts." . . . This doesn't mean that she's undifferentiated magma, but that she doesn't lord it over her body or her desire . . . woman does not bring about the same reorganization which serves the couple head/genitals and which is inscribed only within boundaries" (2052). Rowing as a woman creates just this kind of bodily community.

One of the effects of participating in the practice of *l'écriture féminine* is that it will establish for women a new relationship to their bodies. Cixous describes the way in which the participant will "not only 'realize' the decensored relation of woman to her sexuality, to her womanly being" but also will receive "back her goods, her plea-sures, her organs, her immense bodily territories which have been kept under seal" (2044). Recognizing the physical changes brought about by many early morning hours of sculling on the still water of the bay near her Long Island home, Hall suggests that she is becom-ing reacquainted with her body, not just in a physical sense but also in what Abigail Bray describes as a "morphological" sense—that is how a culture "interprets and gives meaning to the anatomical body" (Bray 2004, 35): "Suddenly one summer I became lean, as my husband said, "stringy, sort of gristly." Suddenly my body felt hot and good and alive for the first time in many years" (Hall 2002, 54). It is not just a transformation from one who "had been large and soft, mov-ing with the lassitude that comes of not enough sleep and more than enough . . . leftovers" (54) to a muscled, sinewy athlete. Rather, it is a process of reacquaintance with a body that is but representative of all of the desires within. Hall describes the moment when her teen-age body "so fierce and graceful . . . so mysteriously and increasingly female, became an instrument of betrayal and sorrow" (41) during a sexually threatening encounter with an older, male authority figure: "It was as if the exuberance—the sheer pleasure in how my body looked, in inhabiting myself—were submerged, a deep underground current still powerful and coursing but invisible, inaudible, unsuited to the light of day" (41). Hall is taught by the community of adults around her that these feelings associated with her newly developed physical body, and hence the contours of the body itself, are taboo.

Rowing as a woman changes this relationship for Hall, and she soon finds she has "become *of* the water, not on it or against it" (156, emphasis in original).

One of the recurring images that is associated with *l'écriture féminine*, and more specifically that represents the "subversive, dissident energy" (Bray 2004, 56) that characterizes Cixous's concept of the feminine, is this image of water. It is *moving* water that exemplifies this feminine creative potential, constrained by a phallocentric discourse that has taught women to fear this rolling swell: "Time and again I . . . have felt so full of luminous torrents that I could burst—burst with forms much more beautiful than those which are put in frames and sold for a stinking fortune. . . . I was afraid, and I swallowed my shame and my fear. I said to myself: You are mad! What's the meaning of these waves, these floods, these outbursts" (Cixous 2001 [1975], 2040)? Given the nature of rowing, water plays an important part in Hall's relationship to the sport. It is a constantly changing medium, and as Hall learns to move through the different types of water in her single shell, she also learns to hear and accept the water that she feels moving within her, what Cixous calls "woman's imaginary" (2040): "[T]he rumble of water, thousands and thousands, millions of gallons, an ocean of submerged energy moving inexorably underneath me, waiting for spring to surface" contains "the murmur of voices, low and melodious, sweet and urgent" (Hall 2002, 57, 98). These voices, "pale faces [that] hovered near [her] bed," urge Hall to "*Speak for us*" (98). Hall's rowing as a woman is thus presented as a form of expression, an expression of those voices within that have heretofore been unable to speak, but will now pour forth "a production of forms . . . a resonant vision, a composition, something beautiful" (Cixous 2001 [1975], 2040).

The "poetry" of Hall's stroke—"perfectly timed, blades perfectly rolled up and squared, dropped in at just the right depth and just the right time" (2002, 122)—comes when Hall understands herself as "no longer a creature of dry land riding the water's surface" but, rather, one who can "feel the boat, the water, [her] body is linked in a rapturous system" (124). It is this same poetry that Cixous believes is the quintessential mode of expression for *l'écriture féminine* (2001 [1975], 2043). In choosing "poetry" to describe the essence of *l'écriture féminine*, Cixous is not limiting feminine writing to streams of iambic pentameter and clusters of rhyming couplets controlled by sonnet forms Shakespearean and Petrarchan. Rather, she is employing the concept of poetry as a mode of expression that is associational and relational, an open system of meaning, to describe the way in which women will write. This "poetic" expression, Cixous predicts, will have catastrophic effects on the phallocentric order: "Because the 'economy' of her drives is prodigious, she cannot fail, in seizing the occasion to speak, to transform directly and indirectly *all* systems of exchange based on masculine thrift. Her libido will produce far more radical effects of political and social change than some might like to think" (2045–46, emphasis in original). In practicing *l'écriture féminine* through the poetry of her stroke, Hall also brings about a frightening development—the ignition of "a kind of emotional environmental hazard" that was "so vast and volatile that nothing would be left after it had spent its fury, nothing but scorched earth and charred remains" (2002, 244). In employing her newfound feminine voice to counter the oppressive control of an angry and abusive husband, Hall admits that she "dropped a match into a well of fuel concealed under the brick and fieldstone foundation of our lives" (244), carrying out what Cixous understands to be "the indispensable ruptures and transformations in her history" (2001 [1975], 2043).

The practice of *l'écriture féminine* is not without its opposition and resistance, for the shattering effects of this expressive practice have threatened the supremacy of the phallocentric order. As *l'écriture féminine* redefines "woman" and all that is associated with the concept, there will inevitably be an attempt to bring practitioners back under the shadow of the phallus: "If the New Women, arriving now, dare to create outside the theoretical, they're called in by the cops of the signifier, fingerprinted, remonstrated, and brought into the line of order that they are supposed to know; assigned by force of trickery to a precise place in the chain that's always formed for the benefit of a privileged signifier" (2055). Just as Cixous's writer is "assigned . . . to a precise place in the chain" of a phallocentric language system, so too is Hall through her husband's attempts to diagnose her with various types of psychiatric disorders. Hall's husband "created a masterful account of [her] devolution, meticulously gathering the threads of incidents that occur in the life of any woman, in any family, and mingling them with outright fiction" (Hall 2002, 253). The "vivid and compelling tapestry of dysfunction" that her husband weaves is an attempt to place Hall and her practice of rowing/writing within a system of meaning created by the psychiatric community—the community whose unquestioned control Cixous is challenging: "Some of his written accounts were typed on official-looking paper in the bottom margin of which was printed "Personal and Confidential: Patient Privileged Materials" as if it had been written by the famous psychiatrist himself, and throughout there was a sprinkling of psychiatric terms" (Hall 2002, 253).

Though her husband makes efforts to contain her by attempting to figure her new knowledge of self—and the creative forms that precipitate from this knowledge—as illness, Hall celebrates the strength of the rowing community of which she is a part. To contrast with her earlier, closed, and taboo relationship to her body is a new feeling of bodily community through rowing as a woman. Cixous describes this open community in her redefinition of "love":

> In the beginning are our differences. The new love dares for the other, wants the other, makes dizzying, precipitous flights between knowledge and invention . . . a love that has no commerce with the apprehensive desire that provides against lack and stultifies the strange; a love that rejoices in the exchange that multiplies. (2001 [1975], 2055–56)

The sense of this community is perhaps best communicated in the description Hall offers of rowing with another—an experience she has when she rows with Carol Bower in a double (a two-person shell in which each rower sculls with two oars):

> We coiled up, blades square, backs straight and braced for the load, heads up, eyes on the horizon. Then we were off the line in perfect unison, perfect intention. I could feel Carol's strength, and I could feel mine. I could feel Carol's balance and skill, and I could feel mine. . . . Carol was experienced and controlled, and I fervent and instinctual—different as night and day, joined in the Race. (Hall 2002, 207)

This is the movement that Cixous associates with the practice of *l'écriture féminine*. In rowing with another, Hall is participating in a community that depends on a motion that dares "to make these vertiginous crossings [and] passionate sojourns in him, her, them, whom she inhabits long enough to look at from the point closest to their drives" (Cixous 2001 [1975], 2052). As she acknowledges her own "fervent and instinctual" drive (Hall 2002, 207), she also feels with equal force the experience and control of her partner. The woman who writes, or, as I argue, the woman who rows, "does not stand still; she's everywhere, she exchanges, she is the desire-that-gives" (Cixous 2001 [1975], 2056), and from this participation comes a bodily community where, in Cixous's words, "we will never be lacking" (2056).

During the summer of 2005, I was an active member of a women's recreational rowing crew comprised of various members of the English and Sociology Departments at Queen's University. Rowing in our straight four, a sweep-oared boat that is steered without the aid of a coxswain, we explored the practice of writing on and in the water. Ours was a bodily community marked by diversity; we were women of differing ages, drives, histories, physical bodies, and perspectives. It was difficult not to note our differences, but as Cixous notes, "You can't talk about a female sexuality, uniform, homogeneous, classifiable into codes—any more than you can talk about one unconscious resembling another" (2001 [1975], 2040). In our practice of rowing as women, we "dare[d] for the other" (2055) that masculinist culture had taught us was outside of ourselves, and in those moments of "swing," when the forward movement of the boat felt like gliding swiftly across glass, we "lived in flight, stealing away, finding, when desired, narrow passages, hidden crossovers" between ourselves and the bodies with which we shared the boat (2050). In the shared act of rowing, one's physical body becomes inextricably part of a larger whole of legs, sliding seats, arms and wrists moving together, and thus each body signifies the "infinite and mobile complexity" that is characteristic of "women's imaginary" (2049, 2040). In identifying the practice of rowing as a woman as akin to Cixous's practice of *l'écriture féminine* added to the possible modes of expression is one that at the same time that it allows women an opportunity to redefine their physical bodies also provides opportunity for the expression of the "ebullient, infinite woman [whose] stream of phantasms is incredible" (2040).

Works Cited

Bray, Abigail. 2004. *Hélène Cixous: Writing and Sexual Difference*. Houndmills, Basingstoke, Hampshire: Palgrave Macmillan.
Burstyn, Varda. 1998. *The Rites of Men: Manhood, Politics, and the Culture of Sport*. Toronto: University of Toronto Press.
Cixous, Hélène. 2001 [1975]. "The Laugh of the Medusa." In *The Norton Anthology of Theory and Criticism*, trans. Keith Cohen and Paula Cohen, ed. Vincent B. Leitch, 2039–56. New York: W. W. Norton and Co.
Grahame, Kenneth. 1933 [1908]. *The Wind in the Willows*. New York: Charles Scribner's Sons.

Hall, Sara. 2002. *Drawn to the Rhythm: A Passionate Life Reclaimed.* New York: W. W. Norton and Co.

Topolski, Daniel, with Patrick Robinson. 1989. *True Blue: The Oxford Boat Race Mutiny.* Toronto: Doubleday.

13

Women Who Ski With Dogs

Grace D'Alo

It's 2 a.m. on a Friday morning in February and so cold that as my car creeps down the driveway, the tires are loud on the packed snow, and the sound reminds me of Velcro being slowly torn apart. This is the end of a ten-hour drive, and the hum of the highway is still in my ears, groundspeed vibrations resonating in my back and legs. At my request, Phil Leonard plowed the driveway yesterday, and snow is mounded at eye level all around me. When I stop the engine, there is no more interference with the night except for Sparky's nearly conversational whimpers. For a moment, I take in the absolute cold, clear stillness. Through the trees I can see the surface of the lake and a slice of open sky. The residual warmth from the car's engine is fading fast. The moon is bright enough for me to see paw prints and a shoveled path to the door. It's my neighbor, my always prepared and warmly dressed Canadian friend, who has thought to do it. She regularly walks her dog and keeps an eye on the place after Tom and I shut it down in late September. Nine other women are coming from Pennsylvania; seven of them are not far behind me in two cars. I imagine them going through border security; declaring to those serious, earnest, young men and women with French accents that they are not carrying any guns or drugs. Or maybe they stopped in Watertown, New York, to fill up on gas or pick up groceries at the twenty-four-hour Price Chopper. I am certain both cars are less than an hour behind me. It is President's Day weekend, and ten of us are spending four days at my cabin near Kingston, New York. Dubbed the "Women's Weekend," it is a feast of unfettered companionship, exercise, reading, saunas, eating, and drinking; all woven together by conversations that only women have.

The weekend began twelve years ago and is now written on our calendars like other annual holidays. Unlike Christmas or Thanksgiving, however, the weekend does not fulfill familial or religious obligations or commemorate an event. It gives us a chance to celebrate being alive, being together and being women. For months we discuss who is going, what to bring, and when each car is leaving. We exchange cell phone numbers, assign bedrooms, make lists of food, check to see if the number of bottles of alcohol that we are allowed to bring across the border has changed beyond the puritanical Canadian limit of two. We plan in earnest, knowing that any arrangement may be changed in an instant if there is an emergency or a moment of inspiration.

Last year, Carol had knee-replacement surgery two weeks in advance of the trip and was ambivalent about going. Like most independent women, she was reluctant to importune others because of her needs. She felt vulnerable; just the words "knee replacement" sounded like an admission of being old and worn out. On the other hand, she instinctively wanted the healing, and hovering, of women friends. When we planned for the trip, we simply reframed Carol's concerns—instead of determining what had to change in order to accommodate her circumstances, we focused on what had to stay the same to satisfy the rest of us. The most obvious condition that had to stay the same was that Carol had to be there. We also wanted Carol's chicken salad, the delight of watching her Jack Russell, Pete, bound over the lake like a deer. And we wanted to talk with her around the table, the fire, and the Scrabble board. Viewing it this way made it easier for everyone to take care of the details. The night before we left, Pat spent the evening with Carol and worked in her kitchen as a sous chef assembling the chicken salad. For the drive up and back, Carol was regally installed with pillows and blankets in the backseat of Jane's minivan, where she could keep her leg elevated. Morgan kept Pete in her car, walked him as needed, and did not kill him for peeing on her leg. Carol may have limped through the weekend, but her spirit was buoyant, floating on a sea of goodwill that lifted all of us.

Now I am parked in the driveway, bracing myself for the cold and the work that lies ahead. I open the door and Sparky bolts out, barking, as if he were an Alaskan malamute rather than a West Highland terrier. His brief ferocity is endearing but not convincing. It is well below zero, and I have to take off my gloves to work the key into the lock. After the incubation of the car, I can't stop shivering. It is only marginally warmer inside the cabin, and I start the routine of bringing the house up. First I set the thermostat to a subtropical temperature, flip on the circuit breaker, and turn on the pump to bring water back into the house. These are tense moments, because if any of these major systems fail, I have no Houston backup team to consult, only my long-suffering Canadian neighbors. With relief, I hear the reassuring whoosh of the flame igniting in the oil burner, and water is only coming out of the faucets, not through cracked pipes or disconnected lines to the washer or toilets. I have to keep moving to keep warm. I unload my car while the house is still cold, and opening the doors has little impact. Next, I distribute sheets, pillowcases, and blankets on the beds and check in all the closets and rooms for trapped mice or other unexpected guests. It is now 2:30, later than I ever stay up at home, and although the chores are mundane, ones that I have performed thousands of times at home, I feel keen and alive. At 2:45, the next car arrives with three women and two dogs—Pat, Morgan, and Jane are the women, Charlie and Pete the dogs. The house is not warm, but at least being indoors is now distinguishable from being out in the brittle Ontario night. Like a fish being released back into the water, I swim down and disappear into the flow of their conversation

Three more women—Nancy, Jan, and Carol—arrive by 3 a.m., and I have a small fire going in the fireplace. It is far from toasty in the cabin, but the fire masks the last grip of icy air. There is a collective and an unspoken relief that we completed the trip without incident or injury; no black ice, no breakdowns or speeding tickets. A bottle of wine is opened, conversations are picked up, and women work in varying pairs to arrange the food supplies, coordinate rooms with people and luggage, and make the beds in a flurry of synchronized commotion. From years of child raising and managing relationships, we have learned valuable skills—packing the right clothes, games, food, and equipment is second nature. Getting the cabin ready feels like a celebration of our competence. The tasks flow efficiently through female fingers without friction or guidance. Eventually the action and talk give way to the limits of age, and we go to bed.

My bedroom is still cold when I crawl under the quilts at 3:30. Sparky makes himself comfortable on a corner of the bed, an illicit venue at home. Nonspecific, pleasant anticipation keeps me from falling asleep easily. When sleep comes, it is deep and dreamless.

Morgan is puttering around in the kitchen by eight, and soon the smell of strong coffee wafts through the house. With my grateful acquiescence, Morgan assumes control of the kitchen and fireplace every year, keeping both stoked and cleaned up. She strives mightily to restrain her enthusiasm for fixing, improving, and rearranging the cabin, knowing that her actions can be viewed as fixing, improving, and rearranging Tom and me. She fears overstepping her boundaries as a guest; at the same time, she wants to express her joy in being there. We have reached a comfortable but lopsided compromise. She gives me useful small appliances—wooden cutting boards, food choppers, garlic presses—and I keep them. One by one, we pad into the kitchen snuggled in shawls, polar tec robes, and flannel pajamas. The house is cozy, and the murmured conversations are punctuated with bursts of laughter. Three inches of new snow fell during the night. The lake looks like a giant mattress covered in a goose down quilt that has no seams. A thermometer on the porch registers the temperature at –8 degrees Celsius. It is a perfect day for cross-country skiing, but not yet. Lingering over coffee and conversation is a luxury too pleasant not to indulge a little longer. Sour-cream pancakes with fresh berries start flowing from the group in the kitchen, and everyone eventually notices the snow.

We are still talking, still laughing, two hours later and have set out a tentative agenda that begins with my leading a coalition of the willing in Pilates.

Trying to keep a straight face, I mimic Mari Winsor's instructions, "Remember your powerhouse."

"We ain't got no stinking powerhouses," yells Morgan.

There are a few women following along up in the loft, but they are quickly off on a tangent that belies the seriousness of their efforts:

"My powerhouse is on fire," yells Jan.

"My powerhouse has been closed for some time," sighs Carol.

"My powerhouse is your powerhouse" Nancy says with feigned serenity.

"You want a piece of my powerhouse?" taunts Sharon with a Bronx dialect.

And so it goes until the routine ends. I am more tired from laughing than from the exercise. Even the dogs seem amused and keep wandering from one prone woman to the next, trying to lick our faces or barking along with our laughter as if to show their solidarity:

"Now, I'd like to direct your attention to shutting down your powerhouse . . ."

Before I finish, pillows are flying toward me, and I, along with my powerhouse, retreat to my bedroom to get dressed. After the exercise, we are fully awake and no longer want to resist going outside. I layer long underwear under a turtleneck and fleece vest. Cross-country skiing is a sartorial challenge because of the intense heat generated. The challenge is to contain the heat one produces but not to the extent that one is constantly sweating. As I contemplate which ankle brace to wear, I sense the change in energy that has occurred within the cabin. Instead of women in robes softly plodding around in woolen slippers, holding mugs of coffee and cocoa, women are now wrapped in layers of winter gear, clomping around in ski boots, ready to take on the wind and the cold. We shift from Laura Ashley to L. L. Bean in less than thirty minutes.

Pat and Mary are the leaders here. They are not only the best skiers but also the best dressed. Mary is color coordinated, correct, and comfortable. It would not be a stretch to say that she looks Canadian. Pat has an aura of command, although she would be the last to think it. Her explanations of what she is trying this year—a new type of protective gel for her skin and silk long underwear instead of thermal—are modestly instructive. We may never be as thin and fit as Mary or Pat, but we can, theoretically at least, be as warm. That is enough.

Eventually, everyone but Morgan and Jan stumbles through the deep snow, down the hill to the lake, carrying skis and poles as best they can. At the lake's edge there is another period of assembling and readjusting. At the shoreline, there is stamping and milling about, each of us hurrying to snap our boots to our skis and get our hands back into gloves. There is a pause when everyone is ready and the silent wintry beauty of the lake envelops us. Without another word, Pat pushes off, breaking the trail for the rest of us. Our destination is the boat launch and dock on the other side of the lake. It is a struggle to breathe and move simultaneously across the open plane of the lake; the wind and physical effort cut off conversation. My eyes water in the icy blasts of air, and I try to keep my mouth covered with a wool scarf. I can't see anything but the tracks of the skiers in front of me.

It takes about fifteen minutes to cross the lake. We reunite where a weathered and beaten boat dock is frozen, skewed, into the ice. The narrow road leading away from the dock is perfect for our skiing abilities. It gently rises and falls, winding through a mixed forest of birch, fir, and maple trees and occasionally running along the shore. Sunlight is brilliantly reflected off the snow. In the late afternoon, the sun's slanting rays ignite a riot of color on the trail, turning the woods into a kaleidoscope of pink, orange, and blue-green crystals. We are the first to make tracks here. Like ducklings, we continue to follow each other through this exquisite landscape.

Our group falls roughly into three ability groups; Mary and Pat are the most skilled. Once we're in the woods, they are immediately out of sight. They will go farther and longer than the rest of us. Carol and I are last—she has her artificial knee, and I have two ankles that have been altered several times by surgery or by accident. I got new skis last year that are the equivalent of training wheels on a bike. They are congruent with my body—shorter and wider—and with my age—more control and less speed. The rest of the group is comprised of average skiers. These women are faster and more stable than Carol and I but not as daring as our leaders.

Although the trail varies between uphill climbs and downhill glides, once we leave the dock we are steadily rising for a little more than a mile. Along the path we all converge again—Mary and Pat have skied to the end and are already returning, the middle group stopped to take pictures, and when Carol and I arrive, we are beaming, proud of our tortoise-like plodding.

"I can't believe how beautiful it is here; every year it just bowls me over."

"How's the trail ahead?"

"Do you like those short skis?" This last is directed toward me.

"Lov 'em—I want to go even shorter. Eventually I'll be skiing on skis that look like cookie trays."

We chatter about the sun's brilliance, the beauty of the woods, and how many of us have already fallen. In this lighthearted frame of mind, Jane says,

"I could just take off my clothes I feel so warm."

"Nude skiing, a new Olympic sport!"

"Can you imagine us with only those little numbers on our back coming across the lake? That would make the Canadians sit up and pay attention."

"Well, what the hell," I said, "We should do it. How many times do we have the chance?"

Hilariously serious negotiations ensue. We cannot ski without our socks and boots, so taking off pants is ruled out. Increasingly outrageous ideas are conspiratorially discussed *sotto voce*, amidst intermittent howls of laughter. If we ski from our current location in any direction there is a good risk of falling, because we are at the steepest point of the trail. We try to picture ourselves plummeted into a snowbank and then rising like Venus on her shell. Many times you can see a fall coming as your skis, with an apparent mind of their own, start on an inexorable path toward each other. When they touch, you pitch forward and collapse in a disjointed heap. It is awkward if not impossible to uncross your skis or your limbs. What's worse is the realization that you are twisted in such a way that you cannot reach your boot to disengage it from your ski. You will have to wait in this sprawling spread-eagle pose until the next person happens by. Surely this would be even worse without clothes on.

A decision is reached. We will ski to the next open spot, quickly shed all of the clothes from the waist up, take some pictures and redress. Compared to some of the other suggestions, this seems perfectly reasonable. We try to execute this plan, but cosmic forces are at work, foiling our attempts. The first camera is out of film, the second's time-delay feature freezes, and the third only has one picture left. Pat gets that one photo—a shot of broadly smiling women, standing in a clearing under snow-laden pines, jauntily brandishing their ski poles in a victory gesture. It takes a moment, albeit a very short moment, to observe that their clothes are piled off to the right and that the flesh-colored contrast of their torsos against the snow is flesh. In another moment, if you are looking intently, you might notice that the dogs look confused and uncertain of where to cast their eyes.

We return to the cabin, still laughing. Morgan and Jan have tended the fire and have a pot of soup simmering on the stove. It takes us a couple of hours to completely mine the vein of silliness this episode uncovers, but eventually we calm down. All of us take saunas, rotating between the two cedar platforms and warming ourselves to the core. For the rest of the afternoon, we keep our clothes on and make choices about how to spend the time until dinner. Scrabble, ping-pong, reading, napping, sketching, and preparing food are the most likely activities. It is not even five o'clock and we have spent more time exercising, scheming, dressing, undressing, and enjoying ourselves than we would in a week at home.

Dinners are a joint effort, with everyone volunteering to follow the lead of whoever has staked out responsibility for the meal. Donna and Kathy, two Canadian neighbors, join us for the evening, and over cocktails we delight in telling them our topless skiing tale. Donna suggests:

"Why stop with skiing? Why not skating?"

"I think you should make a nude calendar, or, at the very least put the photo in the Lake Association newsletter," adds Kathy.

The idea of a calendar catches everyone's imagination and provokes lively discussion until it is time to eat. It is not hard to think of twelve poses, one for each month, capturing different activities of the weekend. The ongoing debate centers on how to tastefully combine these portraits with modesty and a strand of pearls.

Dinner is basic pasta with my tomato sauce and my grandmother's bracciole. Bracciole is a piece of flank steak covered with pancetta and golden raisins and then rolled and tied. It is simmered in the tomato sauce until tender. With salad, homemade bread, and the best first cold-pressed olive oil I can buy in Harrisburg, it is a body-and-soul satisfying meal. There is also plenty of wine, and no one is driving.

Cleaning up, like the tasks all through the day, evaporates in the vortex of female energy that fills the cabin. Sixties music starts bleating from the speakers. Aretha and Elvis temporarily reverse our dwindling energy supply. Dancing and singing continue until all the dishes are put away, and everyone subsides around the fire. Conversations get quieter. It feels like an open, safe place to talk about children, relationships, and the challenges they present.

Camille, who arrived later in the afternoon with Andrea, brings out several shapes and sizes of drums and percussion instruments. She is a masseuse and interested in the connections between physical well-being and spiritual contentment. She took up drumming a few years ago and uses it to connect people. In elementary schools, kids instantly tune into the rhythms and playfulness of drums. In prisons, the percussion seeps into the deepest, most troubled parts of prison-

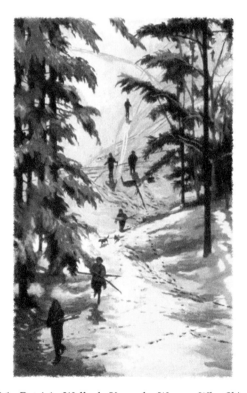

Figure 13.1. Patricia Wallach Keough. *Women Who Ski with Dogs.*

ers' minds, calling them back to a beat, a certainty, a freedom, that is otherwise lost to them.

Camille starts a soothing rhythm on a deep drum that has a warm gurgling sound. We choose instruments from the collection she has spread around the room. Slowly, conversation is replaced with a throbbing that ebbs and flows through different elaborations. I am listening and drumming and imagine myself outside, looking down at the cabin from the hill behind it. The sky is clear and carpeted with stars. I am standing beside the blue spruce Tom planted after my mother died. The timbres of the different drums merge, slightly muffled, as if the cabin is one, all-encompassing drum, pulsing under the soft thumping of invisible hands.

14

If These Roads Could Talk

Life as a Woman on the Run

Wendy Walter-Bailey

I have been an athlete my entire life, aka a jock. Of course people love to call girls who are in sports "tomboys" or "female athletes," thus negating females the right to own their own fit body. Therefore, I think of myself as someone who loves to be physically active and stay fit: I am a runner. I must also confess that I love to eat, therefore I must run. I started running in a competitive manner when I was in sixth grade. I was fast, so I won several races. I ran track in high school as a sprinter: I did not do distance! During college I played softball for my university and I began gaining weight, so I began to run for fitness and weight management. I was also a lifeguard, so I swam for fitness as well, but I found that when I ran I could clear my head and take in nature. I became addicted and incorporated running as part of my lifestyle. Through my life path of marriage, three children, graduate school, and moving from state to state, running remained a constant, albeit solitary, activity for me. It made the daily stresses of life manageable and provided me with a greater level of self-esteem. When I was running, I felt free and powerful in a way I did not feel during any other part of my day. And, until a few years ago, aside from running competitively with teammates and occasionally for a workout with my college roommate, running continued to be solitary. With my busy schedule and young children, I needed more socialization, but finding extra time in my day was all but impossible.

My world expanded during graduate school, when a classmate invited me to run with her and others who belonged to a local women's running group, Women With Will or W3 (motto: women to a higher power). I was unsure whether or not I wanted to give up my

y

145

solitary time (and risk not being able to keep up with the group), but I figured that meeting with other women one time a week would not cramp my style too much. I was ready to take my running to a new level, beyond the 5Ks and 10Ks I'd done in the past. I was ready to tackle a half-marathon, 13.1 miles. I knew I could not do the training alone, since I could never push myself to run more than about six miles at a time. I viewed running with other women as a way to force me to be accountable and increase my mileage, however, I did not anticipate the way my life would change when I started running with other women.

In running with W3, I found a network of amazing friends, women who were intelligent, passionate, and committed to making their lives better through fitness. I learned that this group ran together as a community, and that it did not judge anyone based on running pace or body type. W3 women met weekly because it was fun! My running became my avenue for socializing; therefore, missing a run meant missing out on great conversation. I became addicted to running on another level, and my greatest fear was enduring an injury that would sideline me for any length of time. I expanded my once a week "long run" on Saturday mornings with the group to include runs on other days of the week with one or more women at various locations, sometimes including our dogs. We also planned road trips to races and would incorporate overnight stays that allowed us to develop even greater bonds with one another. We established mutual training goals, such as an eighty-mile relay run by a team of eight women. We trained, talked, listened, and became strong together.

Perhaps one of the most special attributes of the group is that all women are welcomed, and all are valued, no matter their age, occupation, weight, speed, or any other characteristic. Although I could run with varying configurations of women on any given week, the conversations were always meaningful, and healing. Oh, the money I've saved on therapy! Yet another special value of running with women is the sisterhood that develops and the depth of commitment that one sister feels toward another. During our runs we discuss everything from family to politics, to how what we eat affects how we feel and perform when we run. We have supported one another through job changes, dissertations, health problems, and divorces. We talk about bodily functions more than the local colon and rectal specialists, and we all know the areas on our bodies most prone to chafing, as well as the lubricants that help with prevention and healing. Running is not a glamorous sport, and the hours on the road often elicit the deepest secrets to be spewed out when the sweat is pouring and the muscles searing. Above all, there is a sisterhood among my running partners and me, and there is a special bond that I have not found anywhere else. Running is a safe space to share feelings while keeping fit, and we all know that what is said on the road stays on the road.

In our competitive society, where academics compete on a scholarly level the way athletes compete in their given sport, my network of women runners differs. Rather than compete against each other in a race, or even during a workout, our goal is to lift and encourage. When someone is celebrating a victory, no matter how small or large, she shares her story via e-mail, and/or during a workout, and the group members cheer her success. I believe this kind of celebratory attitude is at the core of real feminist work. That all women's victories are supported, not only those who, somehow, fit into the standards of a patriarchal, capitalist system, is at the heart of our mission. In the same vein, when a woman is in crisis, she can count on the group to provide a support system unlike any other. We do not just run for ourselves, we run for all the women in our community, and we provide our money and our services to all kinds of organizations for women.

Over the past two years I have been running with a smaller, breakout group from the larger W3 organization. This does not mean I left the larger group, but when there are nearly 100 women with diverse training goals, we each find our niche with a few women from the larger whole. Numerous small groups have formed; we all come together for large group celebrations, and we are all part of a large e-mail Listserv. When I decided I was ready to tackle my first marathon, I began training with one other woman, someone I didn't even know at the time, but she was also part of the large W3 group. We grew close and told others we were training for a marathon with "a bad attitude"; we would train, but we reserved the right to be bitter about it.

Our idea of "a bad attitude" was more about using running as an outlet for our moaning and groaning, and perhaps to counterbalance the look of complete astonishment from friends and family when we told them we were *choosing* to train for such a physically and mentally taxing event. Marathon training is also a major time commitment and requires a lifestyle change, so we liked the idea of promoting our bitterness to our compulsion. The bad attitude title seemed to stick, and the two of us became the BARC—Bad Attitude Running Club. Since that first marathon we have gained four other members with similar "bad attitude" running goals. There is something about having a title and common workout goals that creates a bond among humans that would not otherwise exist. The real truth, however, is that we are a group of very positive people, and although we love to grumble and commiserate together, our attitudes are anything but bad. We work hard, we play hard, and we laugh often.

The BARC is now my identity as a runner, swimmer, and cyclist. We have grown into multi-sport training, in part to protect our bodies with cross-training, and in part to pursue new goals and challenges. Despite the addition of swimming and biking workouts, we still gather for our Saturday morning long run. The run remains our primary connection. The most interesting aspect of the BARC is that we have two male members. The first male member to be "invited" is a homosexual man, which seemed to be alright for our women's group. In the past six months we've added a heterosexual male. I was unsure at first if this would compromise the sisterhood among the other five of us, but it has not. As a group, we have family outings with our spouses, partners, and children, regular outings without the children, and regular outings with just the six of us who run together. We are more than training partners; we are friends. While the exact word "sisterhood" might not be the correct term, the meaning of the word still applies. I know that if I need help, I can call on any one of my running partners, and she *or he* will be at my side—we are family.

As I have grown older (not old), I have come to appreciate my fitness community as much (if not more than) as any other community of which I am a part. The kinship among my running partners is like no other I can describe. As a feminist academic, I can speak about this kind of sisterhood on a scholarly level, but it is much more powerful at the feeling level. I believe that women need communities where they feel safe, supported, engaged, and empowered. We live in a culture that is clearly "body conscious," and when women feel they have powerful bodies, they are empowered. Feeling empowered physically does wonders for one's mental and emotional well-being. For me, being connected to my body through running has better equipped me to feel more connected to my sexuality and my womanhood. This is a common theme among the other women with whom I run. We hope to spread this message to our daughters, our students, and our sisters everywhere.

While a running group has been my path of community building through fitness, I realize that there are many other routes, and many other fitness options. Women need to reach out, find a network, and build a community through spirit, mind, and body. I view this kind of sisterly community building as one of my greatest contributions to feminism, and I hope that my young daughter will carry the torch as well. As the W3 Web site states, "The mission of Women With Will is to provide women of all ages, all fitness levels, and all ability levels with knowledge and training opportunities in a fun, supportive, non-threatening environment in which each woman identifies her individual sport goals, improves her health and fitness, and builds her self-confidence" (http://www.womenwithwill.com).

My life story is embedded in the roads all over Bloomington, Indiana, the town I now call home. When I'm driving, each neighborhood contains a story, a memory from a previous run, because the roads have become my journal. I am ever grateful for the ability to run and for the honor of sharing the joy of experiencing my body through a community of women (and men) athletes. I hope to still have the privilege of running when I am in my sixties and beyond, as there is nothing I love more than to explore a new city on foot and ponder what I might learn "if these roads could talk."

15

Walking Is an Exercise in Friendship

Marlene Jensen

Walking alone is exercise. Walking with friends, especially women friends, can be an enriching and a transforming experience. I didn't always know this.

My daily walks were quiet—just me and our beagle Daisy. Occasionally our friend Mary Monopoli and her golden retriever Bruno joined us. Those days seemed warmer and brighter because of their companionship and conversation.

When Mary and Bruno moved away, Daisy and I continued to walk, but it was just a walk. And it was lonely.

I noticed that every morning at about the same time, a group of three women walked past my house. I heard them long before I saw them. Their tone was lilting, their conversation spirited, and their laughter uproarious.

Frequently Daisy and I would pass them and say hello.

Soon we started taking a different route through our Vestal, New York, neighborhood, hoping to run into the three women. Many days we did. We'd stop. We might talk a bit. Then one day I asked, "Do you mind if we walk with you?"

They said, "Sure," and that is how Daisy and I finagled our way into what I came to call the Holly Hill Hiking Club. That is how I learned how rewarding it could be to walk with other women.

The group's founder and historian is Diane MacLean, a former math teacher. She has been walking for more than twenty years, most of them with Poeny Liem, who lives a few houses away. The third member of the original trio is Melanie Sienkiewicz, who joined Diane and Poeny after she saw them walking on her street on the next hill over. "I would look out and think, 'Gee, I should be doing that,'" Melanie said. So she did.

It was the beginning of a beautiful and an enduring friendship.

Walkers have come and gone, but Diane, Poeny, and Melanie are the heart of the group. A painting Diane made captures the spirit of their relationship. It shows three figures walking down a nearby road, which is lined with trees and illuminated by sunbeams breaking through the dense canopy of leaves.

Then the rest of us crashed the party.

After Daisy and I joined the group, we became like pied pipers, attracting other women from the neighborhood. On days when everyone's schedule was in perfect alignment, we were a party of seven. And I mean party with a capital P.

Our walks were a combination of a family and neighborhood news network, group therapy, brainstorming, a workout, and, mostly, a special daily connection that celebrated the details of our lives. We were a walking example of contemporary women's history.

We were a diverse group ranging from age forty to over sixty, with children from ages eight to thirty-eight. Our roots are Indonesian, Ukrainian, Slovak, Chinese, Slovenian, Jewish, and Polish.

We talked about everything—trivial, important, serious, and ridiculous.

"What's great about our walks is that you can share the smallest things that you wouldn't pick up the phone to talk about," said Laura Kashinsky, who lived across the street from me.

No topic was taboo. We tackled the grit on the winter streets, the dirt on Britney Spears, *Sex and the City*, aging, real estate, religion, politics, Hindu wedding customs, Chinese ghosts, and Slavic sayings. Favorite subjects included the pet monkey Poeny had as a girl in Indonesia, children, books, husbands, and food—always, and in great detail, food.

If there were such a thing as team Jeopardy, we would kick butt.

The pieces of our lives soon began to form a comfortable patchwork.

We cheered when Diane's son Johnny married. She thought he would forever play the field. We learned about schools and shopping in Singapore from Karen Gustafson, a native of that country, whose large family still lives there. We followed Melanie's son Michael's move across country to go to law school and the adventures of Poeny's son Al as he purchased his first home. Sylvia Marchuska shared stories from her daughter Christine's trip to Spain. While Laura's daughter Lisa was looking forward to high school, our older son Christian was choosing a college.

Only illness, unavoidable appointments, torrential downpours, or icy roads kept us from walking. That hour or so each morning became sacrosanct. Dentists, deadlines, volunteering, and errands were not scheduled until after 10 a.m. The days when I had to miss my walk felt empty and out of synch.

The Holly Hill Hiking Club had no formal arrangement other than letting each other know at the end of the day's walk if we wouldn't be out the next day. One by one, we'd come together as if by radar, then hike uphill. It was a challenging climb, half a mile straight up, but before we knew it, we were at the top.

"I sometimes don't realize that we've been walking uphill, because we're so busy talking," Poeny said.

It was as if the chat and laughter propelled us upward.

Then as quickly as Daisy and I became part of the group, we had to leave it. My husband was promoted, and we would be moving to southern Pennsylvania.

The walking group eased the turmoil caused by months of decisions, arrangements, and changes. The women listened with open minds and with understanding hearts. They were there for me without fail. If I became frustrated by the endless and constant house showings or by discussions with our new builder, someone had a suggestion on how to cope. Someone else would make a joke to ease the stress.

My morning walks provided a needed physical outlet and valuable strength and support.

The last couple of weeks were the toughest—senior prom, graduation, out-of-town guests. Yet I did not miss our walks. Even during the week the movers were packing and loading our worldly possessions, our walk time remained unassailable.

The morning we met at Poeny's house for the last time, I showed up with tears in my eyes. "I don't think I can do this," I blubbered. "Sure you can," said Melanie, as Laura gave me a hug. When we got back to my house we stood with our arms around each other exchanging e-mail addresses and my new address and phone number.

I knew that the bond we formed through the simple acts of walking and talking was strong and true. I also knew things wouldn't be the same. I didn't know if I could recreate that chemistry someplace else.

It wasn't always this way. I had, for the most part, been a solo walker, and in the early days of walking with the group, I wondered how I would fit in.

Laura had the same feelings when she joined us.

"When I used to walk on my own I would treasure the time alone. It gave me a chance to listen to my inner self," she said. "When I joined the group a part of me feared giving up that private time (as wives and mothers we get precious little of that). However, what I receive from the group is equally valuable. . . . It is effortless to be together . . . and truly gives me a chance to speak about all those things that bind women together because of all our shared experiences."

After we moved, I didn't know if I could go it alone again. Daisy and I continued to walk, and although Daisy is lively and charming, I missed the company of other women. No one seemed available to join us to make our walks happier and easier.

Then when our younger son Eric started school, I met Anne Warren at the bus stop. She happily accepted my invitation to walk. "I'd love to," she said, and just like that, my world seemed right again.

We fell into easy conversations about children, travel, husbands, school, and home improvement projects. Both of our sons were in the fifth grade, and both of our husbands grew up in the Rochester, New York, area. From time to time other women joined us, and the old feelings came back—the special connection when women share their unique life experiences with other women.

As I see it, I had the best of situations. I had a wonderful friendship with the smart, funny, and fascinating women from my old walking group, and I had the pleasure of forming new relationships with another group of amazing and amusing women—all because of walking.

Although I have been away from the Holly Hill Hiking Club for a few years, we remain part of each other's lives through e-mails and telephone calls.

Whenever I go back to the area for a visit, the first thing I do is arrange to meet my friends for a walk. Catching up is our first priority—kids, vacations, careers, relocations.

During my last visit, we planned a walk as usual. I met Laura in her driveway, and we started down the street to meet Diane and Melanie.

It was an 18-degree January morning, and we were swathed in several layers against the gusty winds that powdered the air with snow flurries.

The cold hardly mattered. What mattered was that we were together, warmed by laughter and hugs.

16

Marathon

Beth Widmaier Capo

Your familiar voice held an unexpected challenge—"Run
    Chicago with me."
And I, constant competitor, agree, this relationship of pushing
Toward the distant horizon so familiar.
You run your laps around the Chicago lakefront, tuned to
    hip-hop,
Dodging the urban fitness craze, fitting miles in between
    pediatric practice.
I build from three to eighteen miles, through my body's
    durable grace,
Surveying the flat fertility of Central Illinois farmland,
Waking at dawn to run with the sunrise, the sweat of summer
    breaking early.
I chart the growth of corn, greet the park's heron, number the
    dogs, squirrels.
Once I spied a fox, once a camel (in a trailer),
But every mile logged is run with you.
You were my shifting shadow, looping the square, the fields,
Until that October morning when we ran together for the first
    time,
But not the first,
Two pebbles in the avalanche of 40,000 others seeking some
    grail.
The rhythm of the crowd infused our lungs, legs, obscuring
    my shadow
But you are there, earbuds sown, sharing a smile through the
    sweat,
Sign of a friendship grown nearly two-thirds of our lives.

I lost you at the chaos of mile eighteen's water stop.
The last five miles bring internal taunts of weakness,
The torturer's polished tools of pain and doubt.
I chant the names of all my friends, beginning with yours,
And consider the women who brought me to who I was
    when I began,
Who I'll be at the finish line.
Shared visions of swim team and marching band strengthen
    my stride,
You laugh in the rush of my blood, soothe my cramping soul.
Crossing the line, blinded by sunlight refracting off mylar
    blankets,
My jubilation quelled by the revolt in my stomach,
I swim against the current of milling crowd, to our meeting
    point.
You arrive, having finished just fifteen minutes behind me,
Yet you ran with me all the way.
Should we look at this distance, this race run, as summarizing
    our lives,
The challenges we threw down for each other, picked up,
    repeated like the miles?
Surviving each hill and doubt distant from each other, yet as
    connected as a shadow?
And when, the next year, you are proposed to on the beach, I
    run Chicago streets,
And take you with me.

Contributors

Lynn Z. Bloom is Board of Trustees Distinguished Professor and Aetna Chair of Writing at the University of Connecticut. Her twenty-five-plus books range from biography, *Doctor Spock: Biography of a Conservative Radical* (1972) to a feminist manifesto, *The New Assertive Woman* (coauthored, 1975, 1999); to pedagogy, *Writers Without Borders: Writing and Teaching Writing in Troubled Times* (2008). Creative nonfiction is embodied in all of her current work, including *The Seven Deadly Virtues and Other Lively Essays* (2008) and "Consuming Prose: The Delectable Rhetoric of Food Writing" (2008). Every day includes a trip to the gym.

Victoria Boynton is associate professor of English at the State University of New York (SUNY) at Cortland. She teaches in the Professional Writing Program. Her publications include *Herspace: Women, Writing, and Solitude* (2003,) with Jo Malin, and the *Encyclopedia of Women's Autobiography*, also with Malin. Boynton also writes fiction and poetry, publishing in such journals as *Calyx*, *Verse*, *Harpur Palate*, *Heliotrope*, and *Faultline*. She won in 2005 the Roseanne Brooks Dedicated Teacher Award.

Jacqueline Brady is assistant professor of English at Kingsborough Community College (CUNY) in Brooklyn, New York. Her research is on the cultural history of bodybuilding in the United States, and she has completed a book manuscript titled "Minding Muscle: The Technologies of Bodybuilding from the Turn of the Century Machine-Man to the New Millennium's UltraGirl."

Beth Widmaier-Capo is assistant professor of English at Illinois College. Her book, *Textual Contraception: Birth Control and Modern American Fiction*, was published by Ohio State University Press in October 2007. Her research interests include American women writers, cultural studies, contemporary fiction, and the intersection of literature and medicine. She also enjoys running and swimming.

Virginia Corrie-Cozart is a retired music educator, living with her husband in Salem, Oregon. Her book of poetry, *A Mutable Place*, was published in 2003 by Traprock Books.

Myrl Coulter, teaches English at the University of Alberta. Her dissertation, "Feminism, Motherhood, Jane Urquhart, Carol Shields, Margaret Laurence, and Me," explores the relationships that connect feminism, motherhood, fiction, and autobiography. Her research and writing interests are feminist and maternal theory, women's writing and autobiography, and creative nonfiction and popular culture.

Grace D'Alo is a graduate of Carnegie Mellon University and Dickinson School of Law. She currently is the manager of a legal services office in Carlisle, Pennsylvania. She has worked as a lawyer for the Pennsylvania Department of Education and as a writing consultant/ evaluator of the Commonwealth's special education hearing officers and Special Education Appeal Panel members. She is a mediator and trainer for the Middle District of Pennsylvania and an adjunct professor at Penn State Dickinson School of Law, where she teaches legal writing and analysis in the LLM (Master of Laws) program. She has published scholarly articles in the *Harvard Negotiation Law Review, Harvard Negotiation Journal*, and the *Penn State Dickinson Law Review*.

Catherine Houser has worked as a journalist and public relations specialist. Currently she teaches creative writing at the University of Massachusetts, Dartmouth. She lives on Cape Cod, where she works out regularly in a woman-owned gym.

Marlene Jensen has worked as a reporter, an editor, and a columnist at several newspapers and magazines. Presently she is a freelance columnist at *The Daily Times* and *ShoreWoman* magazine in Salisbury, Maryland, and an elementary school substitute teacher.

Jo Malin is a project director and grants specialist in the School of Education and adjunct assistant professor of English at the State University of New York (SUNY) at Binghamton. Her previous books are *The Voice of the Mother: Embedded Maternal Narratives in Twentieth Century Women's Autobiographies* (2000), *Herspace: Women, Writing and Solitude* (2003), and *Encyclopedia of Women's Autobiography* (2005).

Anne Mamary is associate professor of philosophy at Monmouth College in Monmouth, Illinois. She is coeditor, with Gertrude James Gonzalez, of *Cultural Activisms: Poetic Voices, Political Voices* (State

University of New York Press, 1999) and has been dancing since 1990 with the B. F. Harridans.

Kristine Newhall is a doctoral student in women's studies at the University of Iowa and is now living and researching in western Massachusetts. Currently she is examining intersections of feminist activism and sport in the United States in the 1970s. Other interests (research and otherwise) include gender and the gym, biking, softball, articulating intersectionality in sporting practices, Title IX, and tennis.

Christina Pugh is the author of *Restoration* (TriQuarterly Books/Northwestern University Press, 2008) and *Rotary* (Word Press, 2004) and the winner of the Word Press First Book Prize. She is an assistant professor of English at the University of Illinois at Chicago.

Shannon Smith is a PhD candidate in the Department of English at Queen's University in Kingston, Ontario, Canada, where she is finishing a dissertation titled "Masculinity and Sport in Victorian Popular Culture," which examines the ways in which popular forms of Victorian culture, such as the "sensational" theatre, popular fiction, and the periodical press, represent sport culture as contributing to the production of both normative and non-normative masculine bodies. She is also a competitive rower, having represented Canada, in 2006, at the FISA (Fédération Internationale des Sociétés d'Aviron) World Masters' Regatta.

Wendy Walter-Bailey teaches courses in secondary social studies, content literacy, and multicultural education at Indiana University. Her research interests include curriculum reform, issues of race, class, gender, and sexual orientation, adolescents, and dropouts. She is currently working on research concerning social justice curriculum around sexual orientation.

Marcia Woodard is a graduate of the University of Washington MFA program and was the nonfiction editor at *The Seattle Review* from 2002 to 2006. She is a columnist for the *American Kennel Club Gazette* magazine and teaches writing at Edmonds Community College. Recent publications include *13th Moon*, *Kalliope*, *Crosscurrents*, and www.womenwriters.net.

Susan Young is an associate professor at City University of New York (CUNY), where she teaches writing and literature. When not perfecting her left hook, she pursues research in feminist popular culture and is particularly interested in the topic of female identity in science fiction.

Index

A

aerobic activity, 4
aerobics, 68, 73
aerobics classes, 70, 74, 104
ankle injury, 139
artificial knee, 139
askesis, 21, 22
athletic femininity, 84
autobiography, 7

B

B. F. Harridans Morris team, 9
back arch, 97
ballet, 6, 8, 9, 44, 46, 48
Barthes, Roland, 26
Bentley, Toni, 25
Birkerts, Sven, 22
Bloom, Lynn Z., 12
bodily community, 131, 132
body conscious, 148
body image, 64
body image tyranny, 58
bodybuilding events, 80
Bordo, Susan, 2, 5, 71
boxing, 9, 55, 56, 57
Boynton, Victoria, 12
Brady, Jacqueline, 10
Bray, Abigail, 127, 128, 129
Brock-Broido, Lucie, 19
Brossard, 33, 35, 36, 38
Burstyn, Varda, 126
Butler, George, 86

C

camaraderie, 98
cancer survivor, 115

Capo, Beth Widmaier, 13
cartwheel, 96
Castelnuovo, 69
Center Stage, 47
Chernin, Kim, 2
choreography, 24, 46
Cixous, Hélène, 12, 125, 126, 127,
    129, 130, 131, 132
collaboration, 47
communal practice, 87
communal vision, 10
community, 1–11, 13, 44, 46, 53, 81,
    89, 101, 104, 117, 126, 128, 129,
    146–149
community of women, 93
Corrie-Cozart, Virginia, 9
Coulter, Myrl, 11
Crisp, Freda, 45, 58
cross-country skiing, 138, 139
cross-country team, 97
cross-training, 148
cyclist, 148

D

D'Alo, Grace, 13
dance, 6, 19, 21, 22
dance aerobics, 64
dance studio, 8
dance, ballet, 5
dance, tap, 5
Dances by Isadora, 23, 24
dancing, 20
de Man, Paul, 20
De Mille, Agnes, 44
Didrikson, Mildred "Babe," 84, 85,
    86

diet, 46
Duncan classes, 24
Duncan technique, 23, 25
Duncan, Isadora, 23
Dunlap, Carla, 88, 89 note 3

Dworkin, Shari, 7
dysfunctional eating habits, 54

E
eating disorders, 2, 8
Einstein, 44
elegy, 19
empower, 71
empowering, 74, 75
empowerment, 9, 10, 68, 69, 72, 73
empowerment rhetoric, 64
endorphins, 97
Etcoff, Nancy, 58
ethics of teaching, 28
exercise, 3, 5

F
Farrell, Suzanne, 25
female boxing trainer, 55
female breast obsession, 107
female physicality, 44, 54, 58
feminist, 5, 6
feminist academic, 148
feminist environment, 69
feminist pedagogy, 9, 10, 73, 75
feminist work, 147
feminists, 4
figure skating, 47, 48, 49, 51, 52, 53
fitness, 7
fitness center revolution, 105
fitness club, 6
Foster, Susan, 23
Francis, Bev, 86, 89 note 3
friendship, 155

G
gendered and disempowering experience, 70

gendered environment, 69
gendered space, 71
gendered spaces, 69
Glück, Louise, 20
grounded, 97, 98, 99
grounding, 119
Guthrie, 69
gymnastics, 100

H
Hall, 129, 130, 131
Hall, Sara, 128
Haravon Collins, 64, 74
headstands, 96
health, 4
health club, 107
Heyden, Katie Brumbach, 83
Hindu wedding customs, 152
Hoffman's York Barbells, 83
Hoffman, Bob, 83
Holly Hill Hiking Club, 151, 154
Holly Hill Hiking Group, 13
Houser, Catherine, 11
hypermuscular, 86
hypermuscular bodybuilder, 81
hypermuscular bodybuilding, 80
hypermuscular female bodybuilder, 85, 88
hypermuscular type, 87
hypermuscular woman, 81

I
ice dance, 54
ice dancing, 51, 52
identity, 118, 119
indoor cycling, 64, 68, 69, 70, 71, 72, 73, 74, 75
International Federation of Body-builders (IFBB), 85, 86, 88

J
Jakobson, Roman, 21
Jan Todd note, 89
Jazzercise, 68
Jensen, Marlene, 13

Johnston, Lynda, 7

K
Keough, Patricia Walach, 13
knee-replacement surgery, 136
Kournikova, Anna, 80

L
l'écriture féminine, 12, 125–132
L. L. Bean, 139
lap swimming, 12, 112
line (dance), 45
Lorde, Audre, 40
Lyon, Lisa, 84

M
Macdonald, Donald, 126
MacFadden, Bernarr, 81
marathon, 13
Markula 72, 73, 75
Masters Swimmers, 115
McLish, Rachel, 84, 86, 88, 89 note 3
meditation, 117, 118, 120
meniscus, torn, 114
mentorship, 47, 54
mimesis, 29
mimesis in the arts, 27
mimetic, 28
mindlessness, 117
Minerva, 82
Miss Olympia Figure, 86
Miss Olympia Fitness, 84, 86
Morris dance team, 9
Morris dancing, 6, 8, 31
Ms. Olympia Bodybuilding
  Competition, 85
Mudra, 99
Muscle Beach, 83, 84
muscle mass, 49
muscles, 2, 4, 6
muscular, 4
muscular babes, 84
muscular female, 10, 88
muscular women, 10, 79, 89
music, 73

N
narrative, 10, 11, 23
narratives, 1, 3
Navratilova, Martina, 80
New York City Ballet, 25
Newhall, Kristine, 9, 10
no pain, no gain, 71

O
osteoporosis, 114
overcoming low self-esteem, 64
Oxford University Boat Club
  (OUBC), 126

P
pedagogy, 74
perfect bodies, 108
perimenopause, 92
personal trainer, 106
personal trainers, 58
Phelan, Peggy, 21
physical culture craze, 82
Pilates, 138
poems and poetry, 12, 19, 22, 28, 40,
  41, 130
power dynamics, 73
pre-Balanchine, 25
professional bodybuilding, 86
Pugh, Christina, 8
Pumping Iron II, 88
Pumping Iron II: The Women, 86

Q
Quindlen, Anna, 1

R
racquetball, 104
rehearsal studio, 43
Ringling Brothers Circus, 83
Ronell, Avital, 21, 22
rotator cuff, 113
rotator cuff surgery, 112
rowing, 12, 125, 128, 129, 131
rowing community, 131
rowing crew, 132

run, 155
runners and running, 13, 105, 145, 148, 155
running, 105, 145
running group, 13

S
Sandow, Eugen, 81
Sandwina, 82, 83, 84
sculling, 128
sexy muscular type, 86, 87
shin splints, 104
sisterhood, 148
Smith, Shannon, 12
social definitions of femininity, 88
somersaults, 95
Starbuck, JoJo, 54
step aerobics, 64, 68
steroid-enhanced bodies, 86
steroids, 87
Stockton, 84
Stockton, Abbye "Pudgy," 83
Strength and Health, 83
stress release, 75
studio space, 119
survive great loss, 93
Swarzenegger, Arnold, 88
swim laps, 26
swimmer, 148

T
Theberge, 64
third-wave feminist, 87
Title IX, 2, 4, 79, 97

Topolski, Daniel, 126
tumblers and nontumblers, 95
tumbling, 96
Turning Point, The, 46

U
USFSA tests, 52

V
vaudeville, 82, 83, 85

W
W3, 146, 147, 148
walking, 99, 151
walking group, 13
Walter-Bailey, Wendy, 13
Webster, Doug, 50, 51, 52, 53, 54
weight control, 46
weight loss, 5, 70, 71, 72
weights, 6
Wieber, Amy, 41
Wigman, Mary, 23
Wind in the Willows, The, 12, 125
Women With Will, 148
women's running group, 145
Woodard, Marcia, 11

Y
YMCA, 105
yoga, 12, 99, 103, 117, 118, 119, 120
yoga studio, 120, 122
yoga teacher, 120
Young, Susan, 9